Admission and Emergency Assessments

Admission and Emergency Assessments

A Handbook for Clinicians

David Houvenagle
John Schmanski

ROWMAN & LITTLEFIELD
Lanham • Boulder • New York • London

Published by Rowman & Littlefield
An imprint of The Rowman & Littlefield Publishing Group, Inc.
4501 Forbes Boulevard, Suite 200, Lanham, Maryland 20706
www.rowman.com

86-90 Paul Street, London EC2A 4NE

British Library Cataloguing in Publication Information available

Library of Congress Cataloging-in-Publication Data Available

ISBN 978-1-5381-9803-2 (cloth : alk. paper) | ISBN 978-1-5381-9804-9 (pbk. : alk. paper) | ISBN 978-1-5381-9805-6 (ebook)

∞™ The paper used in this publication meets the minimum requirements of American National Standard for Information Sciences—Permanence of Paper for Printed Library Materials, ANSI/NISO Z39.48-1992.

To Charles B. "Todd" Bensenhaver, MD
A man who has been an inspiration in how he works and practices psychiatry.

To Susan Schmanski
Mothered, raised, loved, taught, and shaped my professional career and personal life.

Brief Contents

Contents

Authors' Note

As far as we know, this is the first book for the master's level clinician for the conducting of emergency and assessment interviews. We are not university-based researchers expounding on statistical outcomes from a grant-funded study design that suggests a specific evidence-based approach to assessment.

Instead, this book is based on our tacit knowledge and experiences (and yes, even our adventures) as assessment clinicians in a psychiatric hospital admitting department in the United States. It reflects our trial and error and aha moments after thousands of patient interviews. Our approach leans on established theories regarding human need and interaction that have made sense to us and that we have personally applied in our assessment work with patients. Some of our material, especially chapter 10 ("Staffing with the Doctors") and chapter 11 ("Telling People 'No'") may seem pedestrian, but it arises from our learning curves and our observing nascent clinicians struggle with those skill sets; they are simply described, but looks can be deceiving. To demonstrate and illustrate the skill sets, we use numerous, connected vignettes.

The encyclopedic matters of local and state/provincial regulations applicable to assessment work cannot be encompassed in this type of work. While there are categorical similarities (such as child welfare), the regulatory matters vary in terms of structure, processes, and terminology. Furthermore, the extents of the applicable policies vary themselves. It is therefore incumbent on the assessment clinician to research and become oriented to these matters if these are not part of job orientation.

Acknowledgments

There are numerous individuals who have been of great assistance to us in this project. We would like to thank the very gracious Rowman & Littlefield editors Lilith Dorko, Jenna Dutton, Jonathan Joyce, and Sarah Rinehart for their support and belief in this project.

There were numerous people who reviewed chapters and gave feedback at different times in the writing process. Charles B. Bensenhaver, MD, was helpful in shaping chapter 10. The following people reviewed material and gave feedback: Jim Brock, PsyD; Rebecca Collett, CSW; Kristina Nebel-Hutchinson, MA; Alexis Poore, MA; and Joshua Stewart, LCSW.

David would like to thank the following: First, to John Schmanski for agreeing to join me in this project after I suggested it to you in a hallway at work. You have provided the much-needed energy to get this project done. Second, to my wife, Leslie, the love of my life, who tolerates and supports my ambitions . . . at least I am not chasing windmills . . . or so I think.

John would like to thank the following: My friends and family who acted as a soundboard to bounce ideas off and as enduring encouragers to keep pursuing this project. David, who entertained both traditional and non-traditional ideas and a sometimes-obscure writing style. Thank you for taking this journey with me. My mother and cats, who offered the importance of taking breaks. And finally, Peace Hospital–University of Louisville Assessment and Referral Center, who provided the learning lab to write this book.

Chapter 1

Introduction

The job of doing "level of care" assessments in behavioral health settings is generally an entry-level opportunity for many new graduate-level helping professionals, especially because it does not require licensure or certification in most jurisdictions. While the job title varies by organization (assessment, intake, emergency, and crisis), the positions have the crucial task of determining what level of treatment is necessary for a patient seeking admission and/or empowering them to resolve their stated and observed problems. The excitement of having their first position can be quickly dampened for many because it proves to be a sink or swim rite of passage; the assessment textbook and most relevant clinical course in the graduate curriculum did not prepare them for what they encounter in this practice setting.

Such departments and positions are high turnover in nature due to the lower pay rates and difficulty of the job. While there is a routine, structured interview script for the clinician to use, it is emotionally intense work with high burnout potential. In very human terms, the clinician has the responsibility to assess effectively and efficiently, but patients in crisis are frequently an uncooperative impedance due to psychosis, psychopathology, family conflict, and intoxication. The difficult patients exhibit hostility and may personally attack the clinician as the direct object of anger in front of them regardless of the impersonal nature of the interview. Part of the baptism of the job is long assessments with difficult patients who will not answer the questions and who want to argue with the clinician because they either do not like the clinician's tone of voice or they are avoidant of answering one or more of the questions, making for a frustrating experience.

Furthermore, patient negativity is both magnified and compounded when there is a waiting room full of angry and intoxicated individuals. Patients and their families may wait hours if not close to a day for an assessment. They are already in misery due to a possible plethora of mental illness and withdrawal symptoms, and the uncomfortable wait is lengthened for those in the waiting room, which engenders more negative behaviors. A nicotine user confined in a crowded waiting room without access to their tobacco or vape for hours may face a difficult choice to leave and go to the back of the line or continue to endure the discomfort of withdrawal. Many people who have been incarcerated have trauma issues because of the locked doors and lack of control and can emotionally escalate from claustrophobia to emotional outbursts. Parents who brought children for assessment would rather have not had their children exposed to anti-social and impulsive adults acting inappropriately. The clinician frequently gets to be on the receiving end of caustic patient and family comments that can be personally stressful; yes, it was bad that they had to come to an institution with significant stigma and have their children exposed to inappropriate adult behaviors, but that is an unfortunate and unintended consequence that the clinician has no control over and little more to say than a ritual apology.

When it comes to patients accompanied by relatives, a chaotic family session can erupt in arguing over whether the patient or the family member is lying to the clinician. While the interview is supposed to be a straightforward assessment of symptoms and necessary level of care determination, it frequently erupts into a drama where a clinician is triangulated between the family member and the patient. By virtue of the drama, the assessment clinician is forced to act as a family therapist in the mere effort of trying to get the interview back on track and completed. Such interviews are lengthened because both the family member and patient distract each other off topic from efficiently answering the questions and making for longer wait times for others and thus more irritable patients and their families.

Furthermore, the assessment clinician must demonstrate flexibility due to the various nuances of the different patient cohorts. In one shift, the clinician could start with interviewing a detoxing adult. The next interview in line may be an adolescent with out of control behaviors, who spends a lot of time arguing with their parent figure. Following that tiring interview, the next assessment may be a psychotic adult who fails to answer yes or no to the suicidal ideation questions and goes off on all kinds of tangents. If there is time in the shift, the last patient could be a verbally abusive high utilizer repeatedly complaining about having to wait seven hours to be seen. The variety or diversity is not necessarily welcome but actually stressful for many, and so when the new clinician passes a certification or licensure exam, they are headed out the door to a job that advances their career and comes with a pay raise.

On the other hand, clinicians in rural behavioral health agencies may be drafted to take part in the on-call rotation to do crisis assessments in local hospital emergency departments in their catchment areas. Such rural situations exist because of a lack of local resources, lower budgets, and the relatively low frequency of behavioral health crisis. However, it can mean that a newly hired child therapist only intending to work a regular weekday, clinic schedule is sporadically tasked to go relatively long distances late at night and assess an intoxicated adult making suicidal statements, something that the clinician was not prepared or trained to do in graduate study. Furthermore, the resources provided by the agency for doing the assessment may be sparse and in the form of almost unreadable, outdated photocopies that sit in a secretary's desk for the next time when it happens to be the new person's turn.

So far, this chapter has presented the sober picture motivating the writing of this seminal book on this practice setting. However, there is the potential of great satisfaction in mastery of the work and deep gratification that people in crisis were truly helped by the clinician's knowledge, skills, and efforts. Some people do make careers out of assessment work and are unsung heroes in the mental health profession. Despite the realism about assessment clinician jobs, they can be fulfilling positions.

Another positive note is the opportunity of assessment work as a side job or hustle for existing clinicians seeking to supplement their income and broaden clinical perspective. (David clearly fits in this category.) After all, the high turnover in such departments can mean opportunity. Such opportunity is not only financial, but also can broaden and sharpen an experienced clinician's clinical skills with multiple populations and situations.

Regardless of the motivation for getting an emergency, admission, crisis, or intake position that does a level of care assessment, it is a crucial part of the treatment continuum. Patients do not get admitted without an assessment; it is a part of the continuum that has been greatly neglected in both academic and professional literature. Assessment textbooks used are generalist in nature and focus on treatment planning rather than admission and intake departments.

This book is an orientation and reference for the aspiring student or clinician seeking to conduct admission or emergency assessments in the facility or in the field for psychiatric treatment. This book seeks to fill the tragic gap in the professional literature and provide readers with a theoretical understanding of the level of care assessment. It also describes the necessary interviewing and emotional intelligence skills in managing difficult clinical situations such as those described in prior paragraphs. We believe that this book can be used in classrooms for master's level "labs" and for direct sale to clinicians looking to get into this work. The book seeks to be thorough in preparing the reader with a conceptual framework and concrete practice examples with the common patient populations and the stages of the "level of care." This chapter has painted a backdrop for the rest of the book.

Chapter 2 covers the purposes or intents of the level of care interview. Patient safety is its core, and there are objective criteria that determine what this is supposed to look like. However, the criteria can contradict the patient's or family's agenda and motivation. The clinician often is challenged by that contradiction that presents in the interview.

Chapter 3 conceptualizes the reality of the interview. During the interview, the clinician must go through a deciphering process. A patient can be impaired due to psychosis, intoxication, medical acuity, intellectual disability, and behavior, which means the clinician has to organize puzzle pieces and their overall implications to determine whether the patient is a danger to self or others through "the curve of ability." Patients also have different levels of motivation to answer questions in an accurate and truthful fashion; they do not all want to be there, nor do they want to tell a stranger sensitive or embarrassing personal details. Furthermore, the interview setting, criteria imposed by payor sources, and pressure of risk management concerns all have bearing on the clinician's focus in the interview.

Chapter 4 delineates interviewing skills and patterns. It illustrates the difference between the structured interview typically used in the level of care assessment and the unstructured interview in typical clinic situations. The level of care interview does not focus on spending time joining with the patient but can essentially be abrupt with its blunt questions. To compensate, the clinician may need to use paraverbal skills to instill emotional boundaries typical in professional-patient interactions that include review of the rules of confidentiality.

The professional boundaries are especially important when it comes to the material of chapter 5 and its subject of suicide assessment. There are degrees of severity, standards, and evidence-based methods for assessing suicide. Given the risk management considerations in a level of care assessment, the clinician must be mindful of the risk factors and determine whether the patient voicing suicidal ideation is holdable by involuntary admission.

The clinician will often deal with disruptive, aggressive, and anti-social patients. These patients tend to be loud and uncooperative with the interview. They also pose a safety risk to the clinician and other patients due to their behaviors. Chapter 6 discusses strategies for the clinician in personally coping with and managing such patients so as to adequately get through the assessment interview.

Chapter 7 reviews the assessment of children and adolescents. Arguments with parents or other caregivers are frequent in such assessment interviews because the child and adolescent are not always willing participants and angry that they are there. Due to the escalated emotion, there is the risk of a family therapy session breaking out when it needs to remain an assessment interview, and the clinician will need to separate the parent and child to refocus. Frequently when the parents and children are separated, the children will report allegations of abuse that the clinician will be required to report to the jurisdiction's child welfare or child protective services. The clinician cannot treat children and adolescents as little adults, and there are different standards in assessment criteria.

Chapter 8 discusses substance abuse assessment and its challenges. It involves taking the drug use history, understanding detox symptoms, and appreciating the admission criteria. Admission criteria for substance use detox is determined by scores from the Clinical Institute Withdrawal Scale, Clinical Opiate Withdrawal Scale, and the American Society for Addiction Medicine criteria.

The assessment clinician will encounter people with limited English skills or hearing impairment and will be required by law to use language interpretation services. Chapter 9 reviews the legal stipulations and tips for working with an interpreter in both in-person and telehealth assessment interviews.

After the assessment, the clinician will need to staff the patient information with a physician or nurse practitioner. The clinician must change gears from gathering the information to reporting it in a succinct fashion to a provider (physician or nurse practitioner). As simple as it sounds, it can be an emotionally draining process depending on how difficult the interview was and how difficult the provider is over the phone. Chapter 10 discusses this development of the skill set around clinician staffing cases with providers.

After staffing with providers, not all patients will meet criteria for admission, and the clinician is the one who breaks the news. Some patients and/or their family members will reactive negatively to the treatment recommendation and argue with the clinician. Such patients and family members usually have agendas underlying such reactions, but the clinician is challenged to continue to assess for additional valid clinical information while assertively maintaining professional boundaries. Chapter 11 discusses relevant assertiveness skills and illustrative vignettes of these cases when the clinician has to say "no."

Chapter 12 wrestles with the reality of the high utilizer patient. High utilizers seek frequent and rapid inpatient admission in a relatively short time frame that can even include the very hour of discharge from the same hospital. They know exactly what to say to meet criteria for admission, which can contradict what they have just told inpatient staff hours before the discharge. Some of these patients are disruptive in admitting departments and they are objects of countertransference because of their savviness and demonstration of entitlement. Regardless of the countertransference, the clinician still must demonstrate professionalism with these patients.

Chapter 13 covers the clinician's last step in the assessment process, which is acquiring a pre-certification or prior authorization from the payor source or insurance company. Prior authorization is the initial step in the utilization management process. In some cases, the clinician submits a fax or online request for prior authorization, but frequently the clinician will have to present the case over the phone to an insurance reviewer. The phone call can be stressful as the reviewer can scrutinize and criticize the clinician's interviewing skills and judgment.

Chapter 14 contains our final thoughts on our journeys as assessment clinicians. We discuss a few of our learning experiences along the way. At completion of this book, the reader is hopefully familiar with those common aspects of clinical situations that will prepare them for starting work in assessment or, if already involved in such a position, to be a better clinician.

COMMENT ON DIVERSITY

A few comments are in order about anti-racism, diversity, equity, and inclusion. This matter also includes LBGTQXIA+ issues. Assessment clinicians perhaps encounter the greatest diversity of patients as mental health emergency knows no age, language, religion, race, culture, gender, sexual orientation, or socioeconomic status. While diversity may be an underlying factor in the etiology of patient stressors, it is an unlikely topic for elaboration during an average level of care assessment due to its structured focus. Furthermore, in a philosophical sense, there is always the possibility that patients withhold information in interviews due to their cultural mores or stigma regarding some of the questions. Nevertheless, we hold that there are no unique approaches pertaining to diversity in this practice setting because of the task orientation of the interview; there are only applications of the same skill sets to different situations.

The assessment clinician can encounter the spectrum of political views, values, and behavior merely through interviewing different patients in crisis. Within a shift, an assessment clinician may interview both a cisgender male white supremacist who vociferously adheres to religious fundamentalism and then a person of color who identifies as a female to male transgender and as an atheist. Regardless of such polarity, the consistent expectation is that the clinician professionally and non-judgmentally approach both patients in effectively determining the level of care both need at that time based on self-reports and observed symptomology.

In the experience of the writers, patient accusations and complaints of discrimination have been heard in the complicated contexts of intoxication, detoxification, and personality disorder. The challenge with these situations is that such complaints were part of disruptive behavior, where the patient demonstrated entitlement and manipulation to circumvent the order and in-place protocols. There is the modicum of truth that the patient may be expressing that they experience discrimination in their everyday life during an acute behavioral health episode, and it requires the clinician to analyze whether there is a valid problem that requires an in situ response to de-escalate the patient or an act of advocacy on the patient's behalf. The clinician interacting with the patient making such complaints is obligated to be professional in demeanor and approach because it is as much a matter of order and safety in the practice setting.

Such a professional demeanor and approach includes rational, cultural humility and respect for the dignity of the patient regardless of the diversity and the expression of such diversity. At times, cultural humility requires mindfulness that includes self-checking for possible countertransference. While the level of care interview seeks answers to emotionally sensitive information, it is neither a moral assessment nor a cultural assessment; the clinician is to be non-judgmental of the patient's culture, values, or beliefs as disclosed during the assessment process. We will apply this approach in our practice vignettes throughout the book.

Chapter 2

The Purpose of the Interview

So, what do we set out to accomplish from the emergency/assessment interview? In short, you as the clinician are deciphering what level of treatment the patient qualifies for, which is determined by criteria. Just as with diagnosis, there are rules for deciding if a patient has met the requirements to receive inpatient or outpatient care. These criteria are based on the safety of the patient and/or medical necessity as well as clinician intuition. For example, if you have interviewed a patient who reported suicidal thoughts with a plan to shoot themselves, it is clear the patient meets criteria to be admitted and does not require much intuition of determining whether the patient is a danger to themselves. However, another patient presenting with some degree of psychosis (e.g., paranoia, delusion, hallucination) may be okay to go home and follow-up with an outpatient provider; in this type of case, the clinician is forced to determine if the patient meets criteria based on risk factors, historical record, and the clinician's intuition regarding the severity of symptoms.

Besides safety, there may be external agendas for a patient being assessed. For example, a person may be seeking assessment because they violated their probation or parole and their officer told them they had to do it. Schools will tell parents to get a child assessed due to one or more behavioral events. Child protective services may require a teen to be evaluated due to illegal behavior, risk-taking, or other impulsive behavior. Adults in the criminal justice system may malinger and get hospitalized to avoid a court appearance, a drug screen appointment, or jail time. A person experiencing homelessness or houselessness may seek hospitalization to avoid staying at a shelter or on the street. Furthermore, some parents may falsely claim that their child is out of control or a danger to themselves or others to have the hospital babysit and give them a break. Such parents making false claims take vacations where their severely autistic child may be a nuisance to manage when traveling. It has even been the experience of the writers that some parents have attempted to use hospital admission as "punishment" for a child. The agenda of the individual or parental figure may not be known until after it is determined criteria has been met, and in some cases a patient's agenda may never be discovered.

This chapter explores the ideal purpose of the interview compared to the reality that people have various agendas for coming for assessment and admission. Admission requires meeting criteria or rules that establish some level of safety risk of danger to self or others. The interview ideally has the purpose of providing that information for determination. However, the reality is that some patients and their families have agendas for getting assessed that go beyond the genuine purpose of a true behavioral health problem, and they know what to say. Part of the unexpected, challenging job orientation for the new clinician is encountering this reality and still maintaining focus to determine whether criteria is met.

CRITERIA

Criteria as a general concept is a set of standards or rules for decision-making and ultimately the rubric for determining what level of care a patient meets. In the context of the hospital assessment, the criteria have to do with the treatment recommendation made to the patient at the end of the assessment.

In the United States, the criteria have been shaped by managed care practices. Managed care organizations (MCOs) have decided with medical professionals what constitutes a necessity for hospital admission. The different MCOs typically subscribe to a particular instrument or standard that will determine what level of care the payor will approve. It is the challenge for the assessment clinician to take the information from the patient and family and measure it against criteria to determine if the patient qualifies for inpatient or outpatient treatment.

There is no one set of criteria. Different MCOs use different standards which they consider to be proprietary and confidential. Some standards are in the shape of tables and others are decision trees.[1] Typically, there are relatively few insurance providers that form "networks" in a local area at any time, so it is possible to master the standards. With repetition, you can learn if not master what standards the insurance companies and MCOs abide by to inform how you obtain information from the patient and in making a treatment recommendation.

Whatever the standard, the general order of the system tends to follow the diagram in figure 2.1. Based on the outcome of the interview, the patient will generally fit within one of the three categories of:

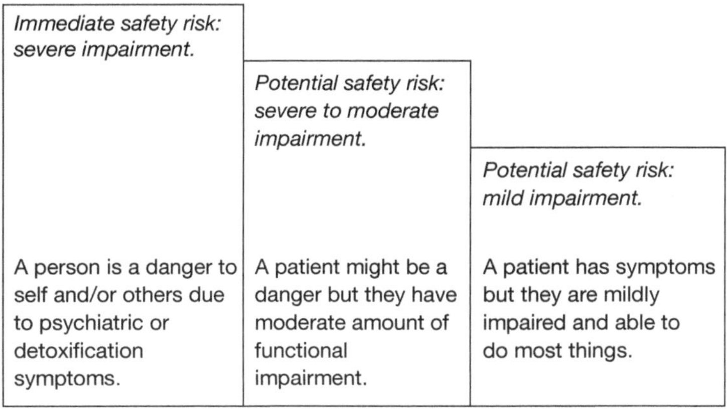

Figure 2.1. The Basic Standard Level of Care.

- Immediate safety risk: severe impairment
- Potential safety risk: moderate to severe impairment
- Potential safety risk: mild impairment

Immediate Safety Risk: Severe Impairment

Safety is determined by its opposite, that being whether a person is a danger to themselves or others. While safety is existential, a patient is deemed unsafe based on what the clinician observes (e.g., drug/alcohol withdrawal, psychosis), what the client or family says, or if the family lacks confidence in maintaining a safe household with the patient residing there. Something may not sound like a danger to you, but to the patient or accompanying family member it may be a danger. For example, parents of an autistic child may have observed him headbanging earlier in the day. Based on the severity of the headbanging, the clinician may think outpatient is best but the family knowing their son's behavioral pattern understand that without hospitalization and medication adjustment their child will escalate his self-injurious behaviors and be a significant danger to himself.

Similarly, the clinician may know a patient needs admission when the patient does not believe it is necessary. For example, if the clinician observes the patient to be intoxicated and behaving in a severely psychotic manner, then the clinician should advocate for admission even if the patient denies needing to be admitted. The individual patient meeting the criteria as being an immediate safety risk should be admitted inpatient for the safety of themselves or others. Some of the major immediate safety risks meeting criteria for admission by MCOs are patients who are

- suicidal with a plan,
- homicidal/threatening violence,
- acutely psychotic,
- severely withdrawing from drugs/alcohol,
- engaging in risky behavior such as aggression or fire starting,
- self-harming, or
- engaging in significant illegal acts.

The risky behavior/immediate safety risk criteria lastly mentioned are mostly in the cases of children/adolescents or individuals with intellectual disability.

Potential Safety Risk: Moderate to Severe Impairment

The matter of potential safety risk is a gray area that may require your clinical intuition whether patients are demonstrating or experiencing severe impairment. Besides the symptoms of depression, anxiety, psychosis, etc., the patient with severe impairment is also unable to work, go to school, get out of bed, and perhaps do daily hygiene. The person fitting into this category potentially could be admitted as an inpatient but may only meet the criteria for a partial hospitalization or an intensive outpatient program. A patient with moderate impairment is typically able to handle priorities but unable to handle noticeable details.[2] These individuals will likely be referred outpatient.

Potential Safety Risk: Mild Impairment

The patient showing mild impairment has some level of noticeable symptoms but reports they can carry on with most if not all their life activities. The person presenting for assessment with mild impairment may be quicker to respond to their psychiatric symptoms than an individual with moderate impairment. This patient may be referred to outpatient or at most an intensive outpatient program.

THE PATIENT'S OR FAMILY'S AGENDA

The assessment is not a sterile event with one pure motivation. The patient and family may have agendas to get some result other than merely determining the necessary level of treatment. The agenda of the patient or the family may collide with the criteria, and it is helpful for the clinician to be mindful of the agenda, if possible. As noted earlier, some patients have agendas of avoidance or compliance. Parents may have agendas to punish children or adolescents. Despite the possible knowledge of these different agendas, a clinician cannot do much about giving them their desired inpatient recommendation if they report severe impairment.

Ideally, the motivation of the patient and the family should be a genuine presentation of symptoms that necessitate some level of treatment. The patient and family are presenting for help because there is the need but, then again, agendas do exist from beyond the ideal. Such agendas range from compliance with requirements by authorities to what essentially is avoidance. Not all patients and their families are transparent about their true intentions for coming to get assessed, but the good news is that the clinician's job is not to be a mind reader.

On any given day, patients will present for assessment to meet a requirement. Schools refer children and adolescents because of truancy, a behavioral event in school, or a troubling comment they made to a teacher, counselor, or principal. Courts, probation officers, or parole officers will send those under supervision to be screened and to be treated for problems. Child welfare or protective services will also direct that children or their parents get assessed as part of care plans or contracts. Lastly, employers or employee assistance programs direct employees with a dirty drug screen or some kind of issue to get treatment to keep their jobs. At face value, these people are motivated to get the assessment for themselves and/or their children to avoid further penalty.

Some of the avoidance is legitimate when individuals dependent on alcohol, opiates, or benzodiazepines face potentially fatal withdrawal symptoms when they decide to stop or cannot acquire any more of the substance. Others avoid losing a job by seeking treatment. Then there is malingering that includes avoiding a court date or wanting something other than the homeless shelters or sleeping unsheltered. Patients and their families are typically upfront with the clinician about the legitimate avoidance, but they conceal the illegitimate. An example of illegitimate avoidance is when a parent seeks getting a special needs child admitted so the rest of the family can go on a vacation without them.[3]

RECONCILING CRITERIA AND MOTIVATION

The actual motivation for coming for treatment may seem obvious, but the clinician is not to be a moral judge nor a mind reader to determine if the patient's report is legitimate. Patients have left admitting departments and either attempted or completed suicide. As a result, each patient is to be taken seriously in terms of their report for their protection, the clinician, and the hospital. The master's level assessment clinician is to be an objective observer, collector, and reporter of the facts from both the patient's self-report and from collateral sources, and rectify what admission criteria is met.

So why is it of merit to have some knowledge or presumption of the patient's motivation? The answer is mindfulness and emotional intelligence. Clinicians should not deny natural, negative feelings when encountering illegitimate assessment situations, but understanding family and patient motivation is related to clinician awareness and the ability to compartmentalize so as to focus on what must be documented. Furthermore, without the mindfulness that some seek assessment for ulterior motives, a clinician may personalize such situations or unnecessarily doubt their interview skills and abilities (Many may dwell on the question: Am I missing something here?). On the other hand, some may struggle with resentment when encountering parents and patients exploiting the system. In that spirit, it will be more obvious when there are patients who authentic and earnest in seeking help.

CONCLUDING THOUGHTS

We will not change reality. There is the ideal purpose of the emergency/assessment interview and then there are people with various agendas for getting assessed. Of course, the purpose is foremost determining whether a patient meets the criteria of being a danger to themselves or others, and thus needing inpatient admission. Part of the journey of both job orientation and professional development as assessment clinicians is appreciating both admission criteria and the reality of diverse motivations for seeking assessment.

The master's level assessment clinician should stay focused on establishing criteria and refrain from judging the motivation of patients and parents. It is surprisingly easy to feel countertransference toward people who appear to be manipulating the system; clinicians are human after all. However, a master's level clinician making clinical recommendations not to admit based on patient motivation is taking a risk that can invite liability and litigation. The clinician's assessment should be focused on whether the patient and collateral sources (family and anyone else) provide "factual" information that helps establish whether criteria is met. The assessment clinician is accountable in the grand sense to the public to perform a professional service that can be measured by accepted standards in the standard interview questions.

Should investigators, risk managers, auditors, and lawyers ask questions later (and there is always a chance of that), the clinician should be able to look at their documentation and be able to explain that those clinical decisions not to admit a patient were made solely on the objective criteria derived by the patient's answers to the interview questions. If anyone is going to decide to decline a patient for inpatient admission based on apparent motivation, it should be a psychiatrist familiar with the patient and/or consulting with a treatment team.

NOTES

1. The LOCUS instrument is an example of a decision tree based on a patient's presented symptomology and functioning.

2. The scales tend to note that legal involvement and/or referral by a legal entity count as moderate impairment unless the patient is a child/adolescent, in which case if the legal involvement is significant enough may be considered severe impairment.

3. This is often a child who is autistic or intellectually impaired who may be non-verbal or possessing poor communication abilities and thus unable to confirm or disconfirm their parental figure's reporting of patient behaviors.

Chapter 3

The Reality of the Emergency and Assessment Interview

Challenges to Validity and Reliability

This chapter explores the reality of the emergency and assessment interview and elaborates further on criteria and patient motivations, as well as what the assessment clinician should be looking for and expecting. It explores the clinician's deciphering processes of the patient's information and the patient's ability to participate. It also explores the larger context in which the interview is conducted.

As discussed in the previous chapter, the interview has the purpose of yielding the information whether a patient meets certain criteria for a specific level of care. In the name of validity, the questions are based on standards of care, managed care stipulations, and research findings (often called evidence- or data-based practice). In the name of reliability, the assessment is usually a structured interview so that every clinician consistently asks the same questions to patients to achieve valid answers to determine whether criteria is met. Despite the theoretical intentions of reliability and validity, the assessment interview is not done in a vacuum. With all the threats to reliability and validity it is incumbent upon the clinician to decipher the available patient information and plug it into the interview.

The interview instrument itself is a dynamic instrument that is shaped by the external forces of managed care and accrediting organizations. Questions are interchanged based on larger initiatives, movements, and trends that have fallen under the monikers of data-driven or evidence-based practices. Organizational politics also can play a part in the assessment composition as administrators have preferences. In the end, the average clinician is assigned an interview script that has been shaped by multiple stakeholders to abide by the latest, best practices, and it should reliably measure or capture the intended information in a valid manner.

However, it is recognized in the larger sense that a major challenge to the reliability and validity is that the emergency assessment/hospital admission interview is primarily a self-report questionnaire. In any multiple research textbooks and articles, the threats to validity include patients not giving accurate information through lying, minimizing, or giving the prompted answers to appease the interviewer. In the assessment context, the clinician is not conducting research, but must consider the threats of reliability and validity on interview results.

The clinical information generated in the interview is based on the patient's ability, acuity, and motivation at the time of the assessment. However, there are times when the interview may be beyond the patient's capability of giving clear and reliable answers. The patient's acuity may be so severe or disruptive that they are unable to participate, which by virtue indicates that they meet criteria for admission. The clinician is thus challenged to conduct a valid assessment of whether the patient is meeting the criteria for some level of treatment.

Under ideal circumstances and regardless of the agenda, the patient is fully alert and motivated and thus cooperative with the clinician to participate in the interview. The patient will readily answer all the questions the clinician asks without protest, and the interview produces a valid and reliable treatment recommendation. However, the patient is not necessarily motivated or cooperative and the clinician has to engage in deciphering the clinical information that the patient is giving or demonstrating.

The existential reality of the assessment also poses a challenge. The hospital assessment interview is not an everyday event for the average patient. It is a social exchange that involves a stranger (albeit a professional) who is asking intimate details about events, thoughts, feelings, preferences, and behaviors. In any other context, such questions can be the crossing of personal boundaries and received as intrusive, embarrassing, and offensive, and the clinician has no business knowing such information. It is possible that the interview questions can pose an indignity to the patient because they are forced or ordered to be assessed or face some kind of penalty. The setting and purpose of the assessment gives the clinician both the license and mandate to ask such personal questions, but there is also an inherent assumption that the patient is both motivated and inherently able to tolerate the resulting normal reactions to such inquiries that include vulnerability, embarrassment, and anger.

It follows in such cases that the patient's motivation to participate is often clouded by acuity or intoxication. The motivation depends on the patient's ego strength to tolerate the intrusive nature of the questions. A patient may react with anger outbursts and refuse to respond to questions that they do not want to answer. The anger outbursts are often related to the degree of

- personality order,
- sociopathy,
- intoxication,
- detox, or
- a combination of these factors.

Given such factors, the patient may interfere with the interview process by being distractible and avoidant, and deflect by personally attacking the clinician out of the claim of personal offense (see vignette #3).

The environment of the assessment setting also tends to interfere with the clinician's efforts to decipher the clinical information into whether the patient meets criteria for level of care, especially admission. The physical setting of the assessment may be noisy or crowded, which can be an additional stressor. People with a history of incarceration may complain of feeling trapped if there are security measures that include locked doors. If the waiting room contains other acute patients with bizarre, aggressive, or other inappropriate behaviors, a patient and/or family may see it as more threatening and dangerous than the reason for assessment and request to leave.

This chapter discusses the reality of the interview situation as to what the clinician faces and does. The clinician essentially utilizes deciphering filters in organizing clinical information in the interview to determine whether admission criteria has been met. Furthermore, there is a necessary appreciation of the patient's ability and acuity and how that weighs in on the formulation of the clinical recommendation. Furthermore, the clinician faces challenges from the patient, family, hospital organization, and managed care organizations which are stakeholders as gatekeepers for the hospital's reimbursement and the clinician's wage. The challenge is that the situation is larger and more complex than just conducting an assessment interview.

THE DECIPHERING FILTERS: THE ASSESSMENT QUESTIONS, OBSERVATIONS, AND CRITERIA

In a grand sense, the admission assessment is expected to bring order out of chaos and safety out of danger. The clinician is expected to be a trained, experienced observer and interventionist who will make a normative recommendation in a particular clinical terminology based on the available information. Available information, as it naturally or socially occurs, can present in a very disorganized and intense manner with multiple interferences, and the clinician inherently goes in with a conceptual framework or schema to sort the information to produce the expected answer in terms of criteria. Such a

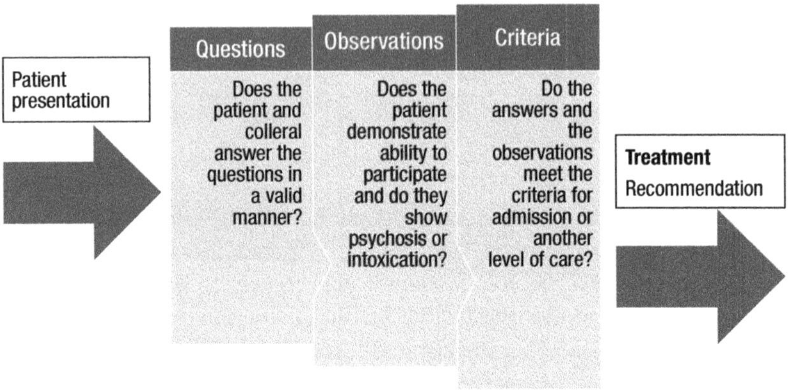

Figure 3.1. The Clinical Filters.

framework takes the form of filters as depicted in figure 3.1. The filters do not necessarily have to be in the order that the figure depicts. However, the fledgling clinician will be focused on the execution of delivering and answering the script of questions. As experience is gained, the clinician will more likely to start the assessment from a schema of first observing the patient's behavior and affective state prior to asking the interview questions.

THE CURVE OF ABILITY

What complicates the interview both in terms of observation and participation is the tension between the patient's ability and acuity that resembles the economic "Laffer" curve.[1] A patient comes to the interview with levels of ability and acuity that can both enhance or hinder the interview process and ability of the clinician to assess and make a clinical recommendation. Symptomatic acuity can end up having an inverse relationship with the ability of the patient to comply with the necessary order of the interview and give valid answers.

The curve essentially travels through four quadrants of ability and acuity. The ability of the patient can depend on the patient's

- medical condition,
- intellectual disability and development level,
- severity of intoxication,
- emotional lability,
- degree of psychosis, or
- a combination of any of these factors.

These conditions may be evident when the patient enters the waiting area and demonstrates aggressive, disruptive, or bizarre behavior. However,

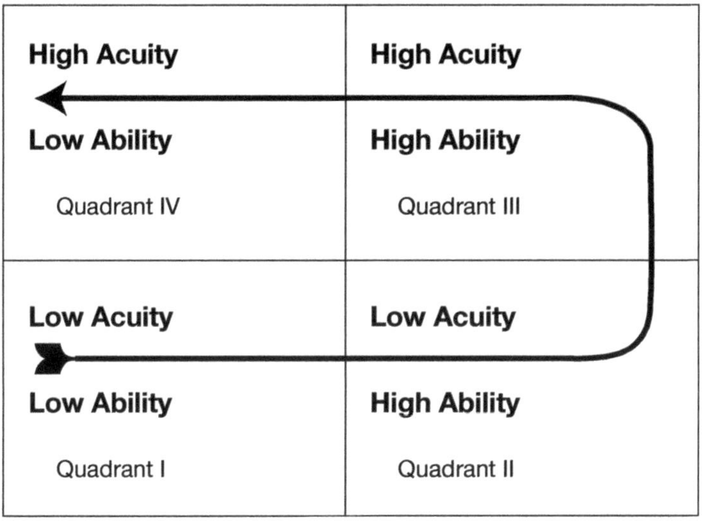

Figure 3.2. The Curve of Ability.

the conditions may not be manifested until the patient starts talking in the assessment interview. The interview questions and clinician may trigger or illuminate the patient's acuity and ability. On the other hand, savvy, difficult patients who have a history of frequent readmission may demonstrate some kind of manipulation of the ability curve by only disclosing enough information to get admitted.[2]

The concept of the curve can be enhanced by noting that there is a matrix of four general categories or quadrants through which the curve travels. These quadrants are:

- Quadrant I: low symptomatic acuity and low ability
- Quadrant II: low symptomatic acuity and high ability
- Quadrant III: high symptomatic acuity and high ability
- Quadrant IV: high symptomatic acuity and low ability

Each of these quadrants have certain patient presentations, indications of patient need, and patterns of clinical information.

Quadrant I: Low Symptomatic Acuity and Low Ability

In the lower left quadrant where the curve begins, the clinician is faced with a patient with lower cognitive functioning due to developmental level or disability. The patient could be a younger child brought in by a family member or foster parent claiming that the patient is some kind of danger or immediate safety risk. The patient may be living with intellectual disability and/or

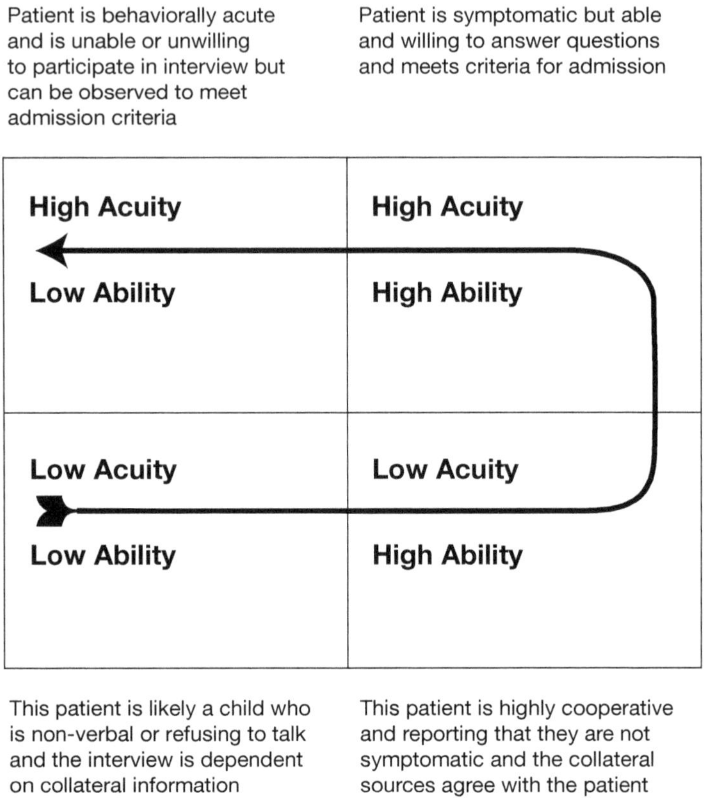

Figure 3.3. The Curve of Ability: Example.

autism. While the patient may be able to give some acknowledgment to a problem, they may be non-verbal and the interview will be largely dependent upon the collateral information of the caretaker.

Quadrant II: Low Symptomatic Acuity and High Ability

In the lower right matrix quadrant, the patient presents as verbally capable of contributing to the interview in valid and reliable ways and having low acuity. This patient is not necessarily meeting criteria for the inpatient level of care. There can be some contention in this quadrant when the collateral or parent is pressing for admission and the patient does not present evidence meeting criteria for admission. Furthermore, the patient may be masking symptomology in an articulate fashion but the collateral source reports symptomology (such as suicidal ideation with a plan) that the patient reluctantly concedes and either agrees to be admitted or ends up getting put on an involuntary hold for their safety. Otherwise, the patient can articulate that they are having symptoms and they are needing a level of service that is not inpatient.

Quadrant III: High Symptomatic Acuity and High Ability

In the third quadrant of the matrix, the patient has symptomatic acuity and the patient gives a report consistent with the acuity or the patient reports in no uncertain terms that they have symptoms. Examples include that the patient openly reports being suicidal, homicidal, psychotic, or having detox symptoms that qualify as an immediate safety risk. The patient may indeed demonstrate congruent affective symptoms of depression and anxiety. Furthermore, the patient may evidence some psychotic symptomology such as response to internal stimuli (the auditory or visual hallucinations being experienced). The patient also is willing to be admitted or can clearly be admitted on an involuntary basis due in part to the patient's self-report.

Quadrant IV: High Symptomatic Acuity and Low Ability

In the fourth quadrant, the patient is unable to give any valid verbal information to contribute to the assessment but demonstrates by their behavior that they are an immediate safety risk toward themselves or others. Psychotic patients may be unable to take part in the interview because they are disorganized, too paranoid, preoccupied in responding to the internal stimuli, or actively aggressive toward others that they are a risk to themselves or others, especially the clinician. (This is depicted in vignette #1.) Intoxicated patients may be judgment-impaired, labile, and aggressive to the degree that they are unable to focus sufficiently to participate in the interview. The patient may arrive at the assessment site already acting in a disruptive and aggressive fashion that to even try to do an assessment is unsafe for the clinician. It is common that the patient seen in this category is

- emergently admitted to inpatient in restraints,
- sent out for medical clearance to rule out any non-psychiatric issues, or
- sedated by injection by the emergency department physician.

Medical clearance at a hospital emergency department is frequently expected when a patient is intoxicated with a high blood alcohol level, has reported a suicide attempt by ingestion of an overdose or poison, or the patient reports a particular medical situation. The medical condition could be diabetes or chest pain. If the assessment is done in a regular hospital emergency department, the patient has had a physical screening that includes labs and drug screens to rule out medical issues. If the assessment is done in a free-standing psychiatric hospital, the accepting or attending psychiatrist may order for the patient to be sent out for medical clearance. If the quadrant IV patient is acutely psychotic with little to no ability to communicate rationally, and in need of immediate sedation/antipsychotic medication, it will be incumbent upon the hospital inpatient staff to monitor for medical issues.

THE DIFFERENT LEVELS OF MOTIVATION

Assuming the patient can participate in the interview as depicted in quadrants II and III of the curve of ability, there is then the matter of motivation, related to the patient agenda, as discussed in the previous chapter. The patient's agenda does not equal the patient's motivation. The patient may present being in the interview as motivated by a true crisis. If there is not a true crisis, the patient can be there by a sense of obligation to a family member. If not a sense of obligation, the patient may be under the pressure from an external source like an employer, court, or child welfare authority. Lastly, the patient may be distracted in the motivation by acuity and intoxication and not necessarily motivated despite having an agenda. The motivation affects the quality of the patient's cooperation in the interview.

These levels also can be expressed in the form of a matrix (figure 3.4) based on the source of the motivation and the intensity level of that motivation.

True Crisis

When there is a true crisis, there is either a self-report or personal admission that the patient is overwhelmed, non-functional, or presenting as a danger toward themselves or others. The patient is truly internally motivated in an emotionally intense way to cooperate with the interview and treatment recommendation.

Coercion

Sometimes as intense as a crisis, coercion is where the patient is forced to come for the assessment by sheer physical means or threat of meaningful consequence. Not all threats matter to an individual, but if the patient believes that a particular threat will either inconvenience them or cause them severe consequence, the patient will present for assessment. Insight and judgment come into play here as the patient may irrationally minimize or catastrophize the severity of the potential threat. This translates into two potential extremes: perfect compliance with the interview or resistance to the interview.

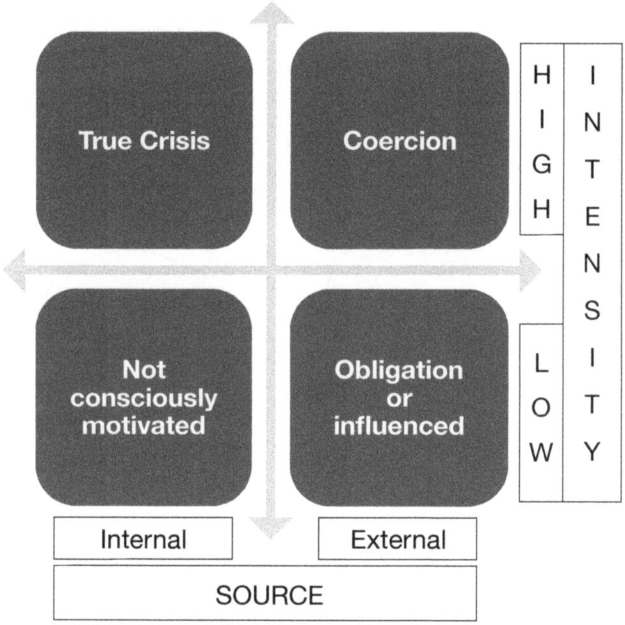

Figure 3.4. Motivation Matrix.

This is the category of motivation where the child fits. Many children and adolescents are brought against their will and are likely to be resistant, minimizing the problem and chain of events leading up to the assessment, and giving both the clinician and parents what amounts to be an angry silent treatment. The clinician is challenged under such conditions to get valid responses from the child or adolescent and the collateral (parent) that substantiates in a consistent manner the essence of what happened and whether it meets criteria.

A similar and relevant parent-child dynamic exists in adult assessment scenarios, especially where addiction is present. The patient may either be under the influence of a substance at the time of assessment or the interaction with the clinician may very well be indicative of persistent parental-child dynamic as suggested by transactional analysis and depicted in figure 3.5. In this situation, the collateral family member condescends or is talking down to the adult patient as if they are a child. The adult patient may respond in an argumentative or oppositional fashion or be passive, perpetuating the continued relationship dynamic. The patient and the family member(s) can be distracted by the emotional power of their conflict in the interview that one or both get distracted and lose some motivation to participate.[3] The clinician is again challenged to interpret whether there is valid substantiation of the criteria

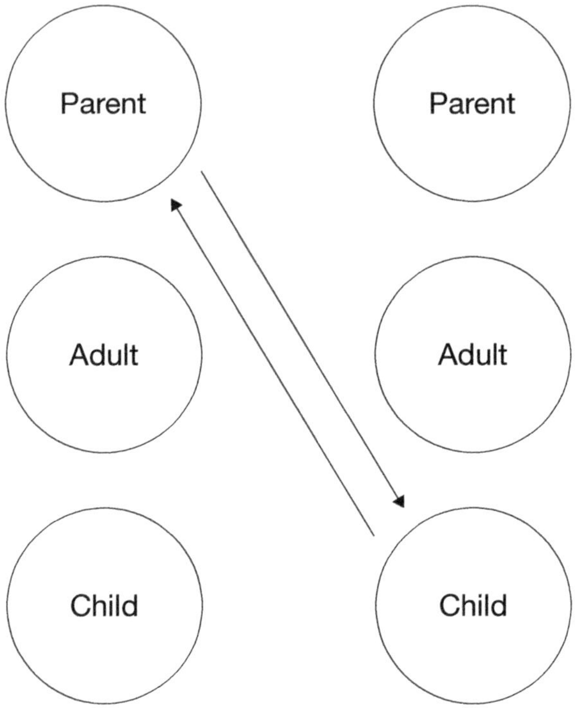

Figure 3.5. Parent-Child Dyad in TA.

for admission, especially when the collateral and patient are arguing during the interview and manifesting a distraction from completing the assessment.

Obligations and External Pressure

Ideally, the patient coming for assessment is personally motivated and desiring the assessment, but that is not the case as the patient can be under pressure or have no control in the matter. Significant others, family members, parents, courts, and employers can obligate the patient to come for the assessment no matter the desires of the patient.

Internal Distractions: Intoxication and Personality Disorder

One other challenge with validity has to do with the reality that many of the assessment questions in ordinary, non-emergency situations cross personal boundaries. A personal boundary is a personal line or limit of some form or fashion. When a boundary is crossed, one or more of the people involved in the interaction has an emotional reaction in some form of anger or anxiety. The basic kinds of personal boundaries are depicted in figure 3.6.

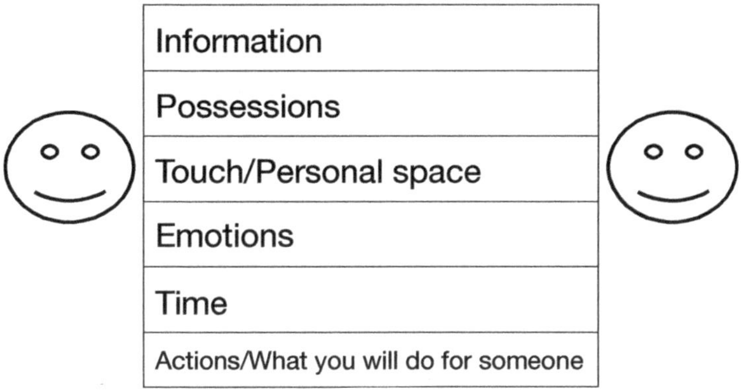

Figure 3.6. Personal Boundaries.

The emergency assessment/hospital admission interview crosses the information boundary. It is asking personal if not intimate information that would normally elicit the anxious response of embarrassment or angry responses of defensiveness or furiousness. Typically, there are compensating elements or assumptions in the context of the interview that can mitigate the typical, negative emotional reactions including

- the privacy of the interview away from the public,
- the qualifying declaration that the encounter between the clinician and the patient is a formal assessment with rules of confidentiality and subject to all pertinent laws such as abuse reporting and duty to warn requirements,
- the orderly form of the structured interview,
- the clinician's professional demeanor, and
- the clinician's professional, non-judgmental reactions to the patient's responses.[4]

The person who has intact ego or character skills can inherently cope with the crossing of their personal boundaries as evidenced by cooperating with the clinician in completing the interview without disruption caused due to emotional reaction.

The intoxicated patient paints a different challenge in terms of motivation because their impulsivity and emotional reactivity are often exacerbated by the effects of the substance on their brain. Thus, the intoxicated patient may demonstrate emotional dysregulation, irrationality, and not appreciate the compensating elements; so, they can be defensive, passive-aggressive, or even personally attack the clinician, claiming to be personally offended by the questions. The opposite of attacking could be the patient becoming tearful and embarrassed by their answers to the questions. One other possible emotional outcome is the patient being remorseful then blaming and attacking the clinician for bringing up the questions. The intoxicated patient acting in a passive-aggressive manner may claim that the offensive questions were not like the last time they had an assessment. All these reactions are essentially an act of avoidance of answering the assessment questions because of the natural emotional pain they cause.

The personality disordered individual may act in similar ways toward the assessment clinician even though the patient does not present as intoxicated. Personality disordered patients, especially borderline, narcissistic, and antisocial types, inherently lack the ego skills to tolerate emotional pain. The emotional pain in these cases is not discovered until the questions are asked. The personality disordered individual can frequently make the interview a matter of personal attack where the patient attacks the clinician out of a perception of being personally attacked or offended (i.e., you're pissing me off with these questions!). However, such a personality disordered individual can already present as loud and hostile prior to the assessment in a manner that puts an emotional and spatial distance between themselves and others; it feels dangerous to be near them and so people move away.

What can make matters more complex is that the patient being assessed is a personality disordered individual who is intoxicated, under the influence of drugs, or going through detox. The patient is demonstrating such intolerance of the interview questions due both to the effects of substances on the brain and the inherent ability to tolerate the crossing of the boundaries. The emotional response can be especially emotional, hostile, and disruptive in which the patient says and does things that are directly hostile to the clinician. If the patient is a high utilizer or repetitive admission, and has developed savviness to the interview, the patient can be intimidating to new clinicians in the agenda to answer only enough questions to get admitted to the hospital and avoid the emotional pain of the interview.

As a normal human being, the clinician also can feel the sense of danger by such intimidation and naturally abide by some inherently natural cues. These emotional reactions include a defensive stance and putting physical space from the patient. The clinician also may feel the urge to avoid asking such questions that the patient negatively reacts to or claims are offensive. It is here where the clinician is challenged to be rational, deciphering the patient's behavior and responses and determining where the patient is on the curve of ability and acuity.

THE EXTERNAL FACTORS OF THE COLLATERAL SOURCES AND CLIMATE

The environment of the assessment situation may also have some effect on the validity of the assessment. The conditions and behavior of others in the hospital setting can color what the patient says and does in the interview. The behaviors of the collateral sources also may affect what is done or said in the interview. These factors may weigh in on how the clinician deciphers the clinical information.

Behaviors of Collateral Sources and Family

When the patient demonstrates being in quadrant I of the ability curve (low ability/low acuity), the value and weight of the collateral sources increases, but then their motivations can affect if not distort the validity of the information. The collateral sources report information that the clinician cannot observe or correlate the patient's self-report. At times, the collateral can contradict what the patient reports or exhibits in terms of

- homicidal ideation,
- violence or property destruction,
- suicidal ideation,
- alcohol and substance use, and
- psychosis.

The collateral sources may claim that the patient is a danger to self or others when the patient is either unable to talk or denies any of the allegations. The clinician is challenged to examine the nature of what the collateral is saying and filter whether it validly contributes to the patient meeting criteria when it contradicts what the client is saying.[5]

When the patient being assessed is a young child or adolescent with an intellectual disability, who is non-verbal or too overwhelmed to talk by the experience, the collateral source dominates the interview. There is a chance that the collateral is exploiting the hospital as a respite or avoidance of responsibility. There is an element of savviness when the collateral provides precisely formulated information so the patient meets criteria. However, when the collateral sources can only report in emotional and general superlatives, the clinician is required to seek clarification of what specifically happened in concrete terms. If the parental figure can only speak in superlatives and fails to give specifics on patient behavior that meet criteria, they can end up attacking the clinician and demanding to talk to a superior when told the patient is not being admitted.

On the other hand, there is much more validity when the collateral source gives specific and detailed information that the patient is suicidal. If there are two or more collateral sources reporting that the patient is suicidal, the clinician has reasonable substantiation for admitting the patient. However, the clinician must often press for that concrete information.

The patient who is presenting for assessment due to drugs and alcohol may be in denial about usage despite the collateral report. If the patient denies or minimizes substance use, the collateral source may directly confront the patient. The collateral may pressure the patient to go into the hospital. In this case, the clinician has the challenge of staying out of the family argument and looking for resultant psychosis and detox symptoms to substantiate whether the patient meets criteria. In the end, the patient can refuse to be admitted despite the treatment recommendation and the clinician must maintain an arbitrary stance toward the collateral that it is all about the patient's choice.

The psychotic patient disagreeing with the collateral source goes two ways in terms of challenge. The patient may have a delusional preoccupation in the interview and refuse inpatient admission to the hospital, but if there is no collateral information that the patient is being violent or physically aggressive, the clinician cannot establish that the patient meets criteria. On the other hand, if the patient is overtly showing positive psychotic symptoms such as response to internal stimuli, disorganized thinking, paranoia, and other bizarre behavior, the clinician can independently verify the collateral information by mere observation. However, just because the patient is showing some psychosis such as conspiratorial delusions, the criteria for inpatient admission is not necessarily met. The clinician must go a step further to clarify and substantiate whether the psychosis demonstrated by the patient meets the criteria of inpatient admission.

Climate

The physical facility, arrangement, procedures, and congestion of the assessment setting may affect the validity of the patient's report. If the waiting area is noisy, smelly, or dirty, the patient and/or collateral may be reluctant to participate. If there is a high degree of security with multiple levels of locked doors, screening, searching, and cameras, some patients with history of incarceration may report an additional layer of stress on account of the setting feeling like jail.

An assessment setting is not always a family-friendly setting and may be either uncomfortably congested or a traumatic experience in itself. Depending on the composition of other patients waiting for assessment or admission at any given time, children and their parents can be exposed to the bizarre, inappropriate, and aggressive behaviors of intoxicated and psychotic adults who might be in quadrant IV (high acuity/low ability) of the curve of acuity and ability. Some adults who are more in quadrant III (high acuity/high ability) of the curve may be reluctant to be admitted out of fear that they will have to be close to people in quadrant IV.[6] Parents and other collateral sources bringing children in for assessment may leave or be reluctant to participate given the appearance of danger of patients in quadrant IV.

The adult patient or family that stays and endures the wait despite such uncomfortable stimuli typically has no options but to do the assessment at that time and in that place. By the time they have entered the assessment session, they may minimize why they are there even if they wrote it on an intake form. However, they may make a statement of complaint of how they were uncomfortable being exposed to disturbing behavior of other patients in the waiting area. The clinician may have to empathize and apologize for the climate but still politely confront about the disparity between what is on the form and what was said in the interview.

VIGNETTES

The following vignettes apply the theoretical concepts in this chapter. They are based on actual admission and emergency assessments. Each vignette will be concluded with an analysis and application.

Vignette #1: A Psychotic Female

Just as the clinician came on duty, the local police had dropped off an adult female who was loud and restless. She was walking up and down the hallway yelling about something not understandable. The police report had her name and that she was picked up on a public street after someone called 911. The supervisor asked the clinician to take the case ahead of the line because of the disruption, while the supervisor booked the bed. The clinician grabbed a paper interview form and went out to the patient.

Clinician: My name is Dave. Can you come in here with me to talk?

The patient came into the room with the clinician, but then started walking around the room and yelling about the people in the ceiling. The clinician started the interview.

Clinician: Can you tell me why you are here today?

Patient: There are people in the ceiling.

Clinician: Are you having any thoughts of wanting to die or kill yourself?

Patient: Now there are people in the wall.

Clinician: Are you having any thoughts of wanting to kill someone else?

Patient: I want to kill the people who are following me.

Clinician: Who are these people?

Patient: Don't you see them? They're in the f----g wall!

Clinician: Are you hearing any voices in your head that are not your own voice?

Patient: They're coming out of the wall to get me.

The patient left the room and did not come back, but returned to pacing in the hallway and yelling in a disorganized fashion. In terms of the curve of ability, the patient evidenced being in quadrant IV given the high acuity and low ability to participate in the interview. The patient evidenced incapability of answering whether she was suicidal. It was noted she indicated homicidal ideation, but it was toward the internal stimuli and thus no duty to warn report was required. The clinician staffed the case with the next psychiatrist on rotation and obtained a seventy-two-hour hold. The patient's acuity necessitated restraints for transportation to the unit. The assessment report established the patient's danger to self and others due to the severe psychosis with repetition of the statement "Patient was unable to participate in the interview due to psychosis."

Vignette #2: An Intoxicated Male

The patient was a fifty-eight-year-old adult male discharged the previous week who had presented again for assessment. In this case, the clinician was familiar with the patient and noted the difference in presentation. The patient did not write a reason for why he came. The patient presented as drowsy and unable to blow long enough to get a valid blood alcohol reading despite repetitive attempts and use of different breathalyzer devices.

The patient fell asleep during the interview multiple times and required multiple prompts to awaken. He was disordered to time and place. He reported suicidal ideation with a plan to walk into traffic. The patient met criteria for admission, but his impaired mental status brought questions of medical stability.

The clinician consulted the house manager, and the decision was made to send the patient to a hospital emergency department for medical clearance. Emergency department labs showed that the patient had a blood alcohol level of 0.250, which explained the patient's sedation. Given the elapse of time, the patient likely presented to the admitting department with a blood alcohol level of more than 0.300, and in terms of the curve of ability, the patient was somewhere between quadrant III and IV.

Vignette #3: A Labile Female

An adult female had presented as a walk-in and had put on the registration form the reason for assessment was detox. During the taking of the vitals, the patient denied any alcohol use in the previous twenty-four hours. The interview was part of a fixed software that could only go in one order. The patient had reported suicidal ideation with a plan to overdose. The patient became agitated at the trauma section.

Clinician: This is a section about trauma. Have you ever been the victim of verbal or emotional abuse?

Patient: Yes, by my stepfather, and by an ex.

Clinician: When did that happen?

Patient: My stepfather when I was a child and my ex when I was seventeen.

Clinician: Do you consider yourself to have been a victim of physical abuse?

Patient: Yes!

Clinician: Who physically abused you?

Patient: My stepdad when I was a child.

Clinician: Have you been the victim of sexual abuse?

Patient: When I was fifteen.

Clinician: Who abused you?

Patient: I don't want to talk about it! You are pissing me off with these questions!

Clinician: I am sorry that these questions are difficult for you. Have you been the victim of neglect where you did not have your food, shelter, and clothing needs met?

Patient: No!

The patient continued to be irritable but readily complied with the developmental questions. The patient began to be resistant again when it came to the substance use questions.

Clinician: This is now the substance use section: Are you a smoker?

Patient: Yes.

Clinician: When did you start?

Patient: Fifteen.

Clinician: How much do you average a day?

Patient: A pack. When is this interview going to be over?

Clinician: It will hopefully be about another ten minutes. How much have you smoked in the last twenty-four hours?

Patient: Two to three cigarettes. This is taking too damn long.

Clinician: At what age did you first drink alcohol?

Patient: Nineteen. They didn't ask these questions the last time.

Clinician: How much do you average a day?

Patient: I don't drink every day.

Clinician: How often do you drink?

Patient: Maybe twice a week?

Clinician: How much do you drink at those times?

Patient: Two to three beers.

Clinician: When was the last time you drank?

Patient: Today.

Clinician: Oh. How much have you had today?

Patient: Five shots.

Clinician: I need to get the breathalyzer to see how much you have in your system.

The patient blew a blood alcohol level of 0.12, indicating that she was legally intoxicated. It suggested an underlying cause of her lability and poor emotional tolerance of the trauma questions. The clinician made no statements of confrontation about the patient's inconsistency about the alcohol use.

The patient's remaining drug use report was as follows. She reported smoking one joint a day. She previously smoked crack but had not done so for two months. She also reported that she had been snorting both heroin and meth daily.

While the patient was still labile and irritable and resistant, she cooperated just enough with the questions about detox. She had a Clinical Institute Withdrawal Assessment for Alcohol (alcohol detox) score of eight and a Clinical Opiate Withdrawal Scale (opiate detox) score of seven. At the end of the assessment, she was agreeable to be admitted.

This is a case where the patient's motivation interfered with the clinician getting a valid assessment of what was happening. This patient seemed to be in quadrant III of the curve of ability, but her motivation to cooperate was affected by her level of intoxication and possible degree of personality disorder. This became evident with the inherent boundary violations of the trauma questions, and she started reacting negatively to the trauma questions.

She escalated very quickly with outbursts that almost seemed to be attempts to intimidate and gaslight the clinician.

If it had been a new clinician conducting the interview, the likelihood of capitulation or giving in to end the interview (despite not having asked all questions) would have been greatly increased. However, in this case, the clinician was able to maintain composure and keep a mature perspective that the patient was acting in more of a childish fashion than a truly offended individual for valid reasons.

Furthermore, the clinician was able at least to decipher that the patient met criteria to be in the hospital for mental health but not the detox that the patient was seeking. In a grand sense, given the patient's intoxication and likely personality issues, the clinician was unable to get a complete picture of what was happening with the client. It was probable that the patient was wanting to come in for detox and said that she was suicidal with a plan to hedge her bet on getting admitted.

Vignette #4: The Adolescent with Intellectual Disability

An adoptive mother brought in a fourteen-year-old male named Samuel. The clinician could tell before the interview that Samuel had lower intellectual functioning by the way he talked. The reason for assessment written on the registration form was "severe aggression." The clinician introduced himself and then started the interview with the confidentiality statement and then asked the patient the first question.

Clinician: Samuel, why did your mother bring you here?

Mother: He had hit his sister . . .

Clinician: I need to hear him give me an answer first, and then I'll get the rest of the story from you.

Samuel: I was bad.

Clinician: What did you do that was bad?

Samuel: I hit my sister.

Clinician: Okay ma'am. I am ready to hear the rest of the story from you. What was the rest of the situation that necessitated you bringing Samuel in for assessment?

Mother: He got into a fight with his seven-year-old sister today. He hit her three times and pushed her down, and she had to be taken to the emergency room for stitches where she hit her head on the edge of a table. He has been escalating over the past week in which he had broken a lamp, punched a hole in a wall, pushed his younger brother down, and has been threatening to hit me. I just cannot keep things safe in the home.

Clinician: Samuel, anything else you want to tell me?

Samuel: I've done some bad things.

The clinician attempted to ask the suicidal ideation questions, but Samuel did not seem to understand them. Samuel had not been aggressive while in the waiting area; therefore, in the curve of ability model, Samuel evidenced to be in quadrant I given the low ability and (at face value) low observed acuity since the information came from the adoptive mother.

The adoptive mother's story was tight, factual, and in the correct time frame; she reported that Samuel had been aggressive on that day in such a way that established there was a crisis. Judging from the record, this was not the first time this adoptive mother had brought Samuel in for the same reason; she was experienced in making this report. This was one of those scenarios where the clinician wondered if this was a way to get babysitting while the adoptive mother went on a vacation. Regardless of the adoptive mother's motivation, the clinician was able to call the previous psychiatrist who readily accepted Samuel for inpatient admission.

Vignette #5: The Patient Who Had Tried to Leave Prior to Assessment

The patient was a twenty-six-year-old male who had written on his registration form that he was suicidal. He had complained about the locked doors and had demanded to leave, but upon review of the form, he was told that he had to stay to be assessed. He was pacing the hallway and had even gestured that he might elope. The time he had to wait between arrival and interview was about three hours, and he was irritable when the clinician came for him.

Clinician: My name is Dave. I am a social worker here at the hospital. I have been with the hospital twenty years. I'm going to do your interview today. The interview should take about forty-five minutes. It is confidential. The exceptions to confidentiality under state law are if someone reports they want to hurt or kill someone, or if someone reports abuse or neglect. Otherwise, what said here will stay here.

Patient: This place is f----g crazy.

Clinician: I'm sorry. What's bothered you about it?

Patient: The place smells. It's crowded. It's loud. That homeless guy freaks me out. I have to ask to go to the bathroom like a f----g baby. I want out of here!

Clinician: Well, given that you wrote that you were here for being suicidal, I can't see about letting you out until I do the interview.

The patient was minimal in answering the questions. The patient quickly said no to the suicidal ideation questions.

Clinician: I still have a bit of a puzzle here to figure out here. You wrote that you were here for suicidal thoughts, but you denied having any suicidal thoughts.

Patient: Yeah?

Clinician: What happened to make you write that?

Patient: Well, I felt like that last night.

Clinician: What was that looking like?

Patient: Well, I was thinking about taking an overdose of heroin last night.

With that exchange, the clinician was able to establish that the patient did indeed meet criteria to be admitted regardless of how minimal his answers were for the duration of the interview. The clinician did not directly challenge the patient on the contradiction and was able to get the patient to clarify why he wrote that he had been suicidal. Using a style that was not directly challenging appeared to reduce the patient's defensiveness.

The rest of the story in the interview was that the patient had been using multiple street substances that included cannabis, meth, and heroin. The patient had done two lines of cocaine the previous day. He had not slept for two days. It was evident that the patient primarily had substance use issues, but he did meet the criteria to be admitted due to mental health issues.

The patient was paranoid and reacting in a heightened, agitated state due to the unfavorable conditions of the waiting area; his motivation to seek help was greatly degraded by what he found in the waiting area. He was in quadrant III and tried to make himself look like he was in quadrant II. Despite the inherent irrationality of the paranoia, the patient did have some valid complaints about the smells and noises, which are often unavoidable in such settings. The clinician was able to work through the poor insight and judgment by showing the patient respect and not directly confronting the patient's contradiction. However, the patient still wanted to leave after the assessment and was involuntarily admitted on a seventy-two-hour hold because of suicidal ideation with a plan in the previous twenty-four hours.

Vignette #6: A Schizophrenic Male with Family

The patient was a thirty-two-year-old male who was accompanied by his father. The reason for assessment on the registration form was "bizarre behavior." In checking the record prior to the interview, the clinician was able to tell that the patient had a history of schizophrenia and multiple hospitalizations in part due to stopping his medication. The patient initially presented as having flat affect, but when he started talking, he seemed irritable and paranoid.

Clinician: My name is Dave. I am a social worker here at the hospital. I have been with the hospital twenty years. I'm going to do your assessment today. It should take about forty-five minutes. It is confidential. The exceptions to confidentiality under state law are if someone reports they want to hurt or kill someone, or if someone reports abuse or neglect. Otherwise, what said here will stay here. What brought you in today?

Patient: My dad said I should come in today.

Clinician: Do you know why he wanted you to come?

Patient: I don't know.

Clinician: (to Dad) Sir, what is your take on the problem?

Father: When he goes off of his medication, he does not sleep, he doesn't shower, and he starts to hear voices again.

Patient: Dad!

Father: Son, I'm just answering his question.

Clinician: (to Dad) Is this what is happening?

The patient's father nodded. He seemed to be walking on eggshells around the patient and was reserved the remainder of the interview.

The clinician proceeded with the rest of the interview while continuing to observe the patient. The patient kept giving his father dirty looks but also appeared to start responding to internal stimuli in the form of talking to someone who was not there. He admitted that he had not bathed in one week but denied suicidal ideation and homicidal ideation. He also denied that he was hearing voices and seeing things. However, when it came to the question about paranoia, the patient disclosed that he felt that the television was talking to him and about him, which are also called "ideas of reference" or referential delusions. The patient seemed to be more in quadrant IV than quadrant III of the curve of ability.

After the interview, the clinician met separately with the father in the hallway. The father briefly clarified that the patient had been acting at home like he did in the interview. The patient came out and disrupted the conversation.

The clinician went and staffed the case with the previous psychiatrist. Given the observed severity of the patient's psychosis (responding to internal stimuli and referential delusions), the psychiatrist issued an order to admit the patient on a seventy-two-hour hold.

This was a case where there was a dynamic of emotional chaos between the patient and his father. While he was an adult, his father still was talking about him in a parental fashion, but then out of his paranoia, the patient angrily pressured his father to be quiet. This was a case where the symptomology was strong enough for the clinician to make valid observations despite the paranoid patient's efforts to silence his father.

Vignette #7: The Aggressive High Utilizer

The patient was a thirty-five-year-old female who was known as a frequent flyer in the department. She came in and wrote one word on her registration form: "Suicidal!" She laid on the floor and covered herself up. When it came time for the assessment, the patient refused to come in for the interview.

Clinician: Ms. Jean, it's time for your assessment.

Patient: I'M SUICIDAL! I'M HEARING VOICES! THAT'S ALL YOU NEED TO KNOW!

Clinician: Not quite. I have to ask some other questions.

Patient: I TOLD YOU ALL I AM GOING TO TELL YOU!

Despite the patient's likely malingering, this was enough information to establish criteria to be admitted to the hospital. She was demonstrating enough ability and motivation (quadrant III) to say she had the acuity to be admitted. She was just not motivated to take part in the whole interview, and she was savvy on how to give just enough information to get admitted by presenting as hostile and intimidating.

Vignette #8: The Angry Adolescent

The patient was a fourteen-year-old female who was brought in by her mother. The report on the registration form was: "Out of Control and Severe Aggression." Prior to the assessment, a code was called where the mother and the patient had to be separated. The mother was being kept in a different waiting area from the patient. The patient also had made a gesture to elope from the department. The patient had been observed to be constantly on her phone texting and reading texts up until the time of the interview. The clinician was able to review the record prior to the assessment and see that the patient had a history of multiple hospitalizations for aggression. The record also showed that the patient had a history of poor medication compliance and had already started using substances. The clinician started the interview with both the mother and patient in the interview room and quickly found there was the need to separate them again almost immediately.

Mother: You have got to do something with my daughter. I just can't take her attitude anymore. She is not taking her medicine and she is out screwing anything with a d—k.

Patient: Yeah, my mom is one to talk. She leaves her bedroom unlocked and sometimes the door is open, and I see what kind of ugly and nasty men she f—ks! It is just nasty. When she finally keeps the door closed, she screams so loud that the neighbors down the street can hear her f---king!

Clinician: Well, with that, let me introduce myself first. I'm Dave. I've been with the hospital twenty years, and I am going to do the assessment. I also need to say that this is a confidential interview but the law says I have to report abuse and neglect to protective services and if someone says they are going to hurt or kill someone I have to make what is called a duty to warn report. Otherwise, what said here will stay here. (To the patient) Why did your mother bring you here?

Patient: (Shrugs and does not answer)

Clinician: Okay ma'am. What happened that you needed to bring your daughter back in for assessment?

Mother: She's not taking her medication. She has been gone for the past month, and she has not attended school. I'm sure she has been doing drugs, and I'm pretty sure she is having unprotected sex. When she finally came home today and I tried to get her in the car to come here, she hit me and said that she was going to send her gang to kill me!

Patient: Quit your lying on me!

At this, the patient stood up and got in the mother's personal space. The clinician had to press the code transponder for assistance. A code team arrived, and the patient was escorted back out to the waiting area.

After a few deep breaths, the clinician met with the patient's mother to get the details in a less-emotional fashion. The mother repeated the information that since the patient had last been in the hospital three months ago, she stopped taking her medication and had eloped from the home. The clinician followed up on the mother's statement of the patient engaging in unprotected sex, and the mother responded that she really did not know if the patient was, but she had searched the patient's room and found condoms and found on the cloud that the patient had previously engaged in sexting. The mother added that was part of the patient hitting her today when the mother tried to take the patient's phone and get her into the car.

The clinician then decided to interview the patient out in the hallway apart from her mother. The patient denied suicidal ideation but reported that she did want to hit her mother. The patient admitted that she had not taken her medication nor did the patient want to take her medication. When asked about not having been at school for the past two months, the patient looked at the clinician and said "So?"

The clinician called the previous psychiatrist who accepted the patient for inpatient. When it was time to go to the unit, the patient had to be escorted by the code team again who forcibly had to get the patient's phone as part of the admission process because she would not give it up.

This was a case of chaotic enmeshment between the mother and patient. They demonstrated an intense amount of anger and poor boundaries. They both seemed to weaponize each other's dirty laundry in a way that obstructed the clinician's conducting the interview and that required separating the mother and patient.

When the clinician separated the patient and parent, he was able to get valid information that established criteria for admission. Isolating the patient from the mother also suggested that the patient fit in quadrant III (high acuity and high ability) despite the patient's poor motivation.

CONCLUDING THOUGHTS

The assessment interview with all the thought that has gone into it has assumptions:

1. It will be an orderly process;
2. All patients will be willing to participate;
3. All patients are motivated to participate; AND (capitalizing intended)
4. All the puzzle pieces to make an assessment will be there.

With time an assessment clinician will encounter a patient who

- refuses to talk,
- be unable to talk, or
- be incapable of understanding the questions.

Furthermore, there will be otherwise capable but uncooperative patients who are angry, unpleasant, and rude due to the misery of detox symptoms or personality disorder traits. Their irritability can be exacerbated because they have poor distress tolerance. This chapter has suggested some frameworks and strategies for when these interviews are piles of puzzle pieces.

The curve of ability framework recognizes that patients present for assessment with different levels of acuity and ability to participate. The woman in vignette #1 was too psychotic (probably from using meth and not sleeping for several days) to able to say whether she was suicidal. Even though he said that he was suicidal, it turned out that the man in vignette #2 was dangerously intoxicated as he was repeatedly falling asleep and did not seem to have the air capacity to blow a blood alcohol level. However, the kid in vignette #4 would at face value fit in quadrant #1 with his intellectual disability and low observed acuity, but the adoptive mother's story provided all the "details" of why there was a crisis. To cut to the chase, the main message of the curve of ability is that barring medical problems and intellectual disability, an inability to participate in an assessment generally equals that criteria for admission are met because a patient cannot answer whether they are suicidal or homicidal.

However, it is not always about the ability as motivation can play into the puzzle. There is an emotional *rubber that meets the road* when it comes to the interview, because the questions are supposed to elicit the disclosure of personal information. When some patients hear questions that trigger their painful trauma memories, secrets, shame, and embarrassments, they can put up emotional walls. The patient's pain can get compounded if they are intoxicated, detoxing, or are maybe even off their medication. The female in vignette #3 appeared to be miserable already from detox and probably had personality disorder traits, and acted the way she did in the interview because it felt like someone rubbing salt in her emotional wounds. The male in vignette #5 also was going through detox and his symptoms made dealing with the environment of the waiting room unbearable that he lost motivation to be assessed, almost bolted from the department, and gave the clinician an ear full. The female in vignette #7 presented as a treatment-savvy manipulative individual who wanted to be admitted but used a mixture of intimidation and refusal to avoid rehashing the assessment information she had provided numerous times. Such patients with low motivation will not give all the information needed for a complete assessment and so the clinician must ask whether there is enough to establish the criteria that the patient is a danger to themselves or others.

Lastly, there can be some family conflict that can interfere with the clinician getting a valid picture of the problem. Vignette #8 was an example of this when the patient and her mother immediately started arguing in an intensely embarrassing way from the moment they got into the admitting department to wait, and then carried on the argument when the clinician tried to start the interview. There was probably some truth to the mother and patient's mutual criticisms of the other's sexual behaviors, but it was irrelevant to the reason for bringing the patient to the hospital.

In the end, despite this chapter's quest to understand what is valid and the threats to validity, the true picture will not always be found. A patient's or family member's true agenda can remain hidden despite the detailed information they give about symptoms and problems. In the end, the clinician's job is not to be a mind reader or a psychic as to whether the parent or patient is lying, but to assess if there is indication that someone needs to be admitted to the hospital for safety.

NOTES

1. The "Laffer" curve is an economic theory used to support "supply-side" economics advocating for less taxation. It suggested that higher tax assessments ended up in less tax revenue because taxation inhibited economic growth and shrunk the overall economic pie. According to Laffer, lower tax assessment will end up in higher tax revenue and eventually end up in more tax revenue because there will be more growth, a larger economic pie, and the piece of that pie will be more revenue. The adaptation of the Laffer curve for this purpose is not an endorsement of this economic view. A. B. Laffer, 2004, "The laffer curve: Past, present and future," Article No. 1765, The Heritage Foundation Publications, 1–16.
2. Patients who are high utilizers, malingers, or frequent readmissions develop experience of the admission process and appreciation of how to manipulate it to say as little as necessary to get admitted. They also can become aggressive or disruptive in waiting areas to create crises and get expedited admissions to units.
3. At times, a patient may come in for assessment and not evidence criteria for any services. After the patient leaves, a family member or collateral may call an admission department in a state of anger complaining that the patient had been suicidal or minimizing the problem (this is depicted in vignette #6 in chapter 11). In a family context, coercion is often only effective if the family member is physically present to give timely, collateral information to the clinician during the assessment.
4. Sometimes during the interview, the patient may disclose information that calls for a legitimate, empathetic response by the clinician to the patient when the patient discloses trauma or tragedy and then starts crying or having some other emotional reaction.
5. Like stated in endnote #3, some collateral reports are made after the patient interview and after the patient has left the facility. The collateral may complain that the patient had been suicidal and should have not been let out of the facility. The clinician may have to set limits with the collateral source that includes suggesting that they bring the patient back and participate in the assessment or seek an involuntary commitment (this is depicted in vignette #6 in chapter 11).
6. They are already in a vulnerable situation with a high level of anxiety and such other patients exacerbate the sense of danger.

Chapter 4

Interviewing Skills and Patterns

The assessment interview is not merely going into a room and having a conversation with a patient. It is an intentional, professional-client encounter with intended results. However, it has the potential of being an intense, emotional encounter for both the patient and the clinician.

As touched on in the previous chapter, the subject matter of the assessment is personal and intimate. Personal information as such is tied to emotions. Emotional triggers and reactions help a person protect boundaries. If asked a personal question by someone who is not respected, trusted, or otherwise has been given the right to know, an individual's emotional response is likely to be that of anxiety or anger. The anxious response may be embarrassment or silence. The angry responses can include defensiveness, hostility, or even a personal attack on the inquirer. A patient who is demonstrating irrationality may have emotional responses that disrupt the interview and impede the clinician's job.

Thus, while it has the purpose of being clinical and benign, the assessment interview can push emotional buttons. There are subjects that are more sensitive to people like substance use, sex, and trauma. When the clinician is asking these questions, there is the risk that the patient will bring up painful memories or thoughts of personal shame. Many patients will react to some sections by crying. Some will become defensive or combative during the drug use and trauma histories. Others will just refuse to answer. Individuals who use substances may be avoidant by claiming the interview did not have these questions as the last time or by trying to rush the clinician out of a claim of physical discomfort. Intoxication or detox symptoms can amplify such emotional reactions, and the clinician has several potential challenges to complete the tasks of the interview.[1]

While it can be assumed that patients have an agenda for the interview, their emotional states can impede and disrupt the interview. Higher levels of emotions can mean higher levels of impulsivity. The clinician does not expect to go into an interview to be personally or physically attacked by a patient, but it can happen. It is a typical assumption that the patient (and perhaps present collateral source) will be motivated and cooperative with all the questions within a reasonable amount of time. Of course, the exceptions do occur, and patients can become argumentative with clinicians instead of answering the questions; the clinician is expected to have the interview skills to work through the emotion and complete the assessment.

This chapter covers relevant interview skills necessary for the emergency and assessment interview. It will discuss the nature of the structured interview and the necessary joining with the patient and family to set the emotional tone. It will cover some skills and strategies to work through difficult and potentially disruptive emotional interview situations.

THE STRUCTURED VERSUS THE UNSTRUCTURED INTERVIEW PATTERN

There are two different types of interviews: the structured and the unstructured. The unstructured interview is a conversation between a clinician and patient that does not have a planned pattern. It is a natural exchange based on what the patient and clinician both desire to discuss. The unstructured interview is also dependent on the relationship between the clinician and patient and how motivated each party is to participate. On the other hand, the structured interview is a predetermined task-oriented script of specific questions. The clinician has the job of getting through the structured interview as opposed to simultaneously joining with the patient and acquiring the pertinent clinical information in the context of a therapeutic relationship.

The unstructured interview very much depends on the sense of position, power, and compliance for the quality of information. For example, a physician has the authoritative and expert position to interview a patient, and the patient is expected to answer the physician's questions. A master's level assessment clinician may not gain the same level of recognition and cooperation of the patient if the patient is not interested in talking to them as much as they might be to a doctor who can prescribe medication.[2]

The quality of the unstructured interview is also dependent on the inherent skill and experience of the clinician. The more a clinician has routinely done an unstructured interview, the more likely the clinician will gain all the necessary information required in an assessment. Regardless of the skill, there is the likelihood that necessary information is going to be missing.

In research terms, the unstructured interview lacks reliability because it is unlikely to yield the same information from clinician to clinician regardless of experience.

This is where the structured interview comes in as more reliable because different clinicians doing the same interview are expected to get similar results or outcomes. The results are expected to be answers that determine whether criteria for admission are met; patients evidencing immediate safety risk are referred for admission. There will still be individual differences in style and approach from clinician to clinician, but the essential questions will consistently get asked and hopefully answered by the patient.

JOINING WITH THE PATIENT: FORMALITY, TONE OF VOICE, AND CONFIDENCE

As stated elsewhere, the assessment clinician does not have to join with the patient in the same manner as required by an outpatient therapist. The assessment clinician is only to meet with a patient one time compared to multiple times by the outpatient therapist. It serves to mention here that the task of the assessment clinician is not to uncover all the underlying factors to the symptoms, but only the necessary information to establish level of care criteria. The outpatient therapist who renders the treatment will need to make a more extensive attempt to join with the patient. The assessment clinician has a task to achieve in a short period of time, and a patient is reasonably expected to cooperate.[3] Nevertheless, there must be some kind of joining with a patient to get them to cooperate with the formal task at hand.

In terms of joining between the patient and the clinician, it seems valuable to build some level of rapport. Although this is not a therapy session where rapport building is more practical, there are a few strategies that can be used to make a bond/connection. For example:

- Complimenting the individual for seeking help
- Exhibiting active listening
- Empathetic comments and facial expressions (e.g., "Wow, that must have been awful")
- Allowing the patient the opportunity to vent
- Giving the patient a moment to regroup after expressing something traumatic
- Offering a snack or water to the patient

Essentially any medical emergency first responders and medical professionals use formality as a demeanor that compensates for the high level of emotion. Medical professionals (including physicians) introduce themselves by title and last name to the patient, which invokes expertise and authority to gain a patient's cooperation so as to conduct a valid examination and render an effective treatment to resolve a patient's medical emergency.[4] A medical professional also will call adult patients by titles such as "Mr." or "Ms.,"[5] which in reality compensates for the patient's possible vulnerability, defensiveness, and embarrassment that would be expected at the normal intrusiveness of asking personal questions. Formality is a necessary element in emergencies.

Whether the patient is mindful of it or not, formality is a paraverbal boundary that can supply a subtle sense of safety and security to the patient, which should result in some trust by the clinician as evidenced as cooperation. As discussed in the previous chapter, the emergency medical encounter and assessment is an emotional transaction that can be examined in terms of Berne's transactional analysis.[6] In Berne's framework, people have emotional exchanges on three levels of ego states: parent, adult, and child (figure 4.1). The child level is impulsive and emotional. The parent level is caretaking, controlling, and (for the purposes of the interview) judgmental-sounding. The adult state is a calm, rational, factual level. The clinician needs to operate and remain at the adult level regardless of the patient's emotional reactions.

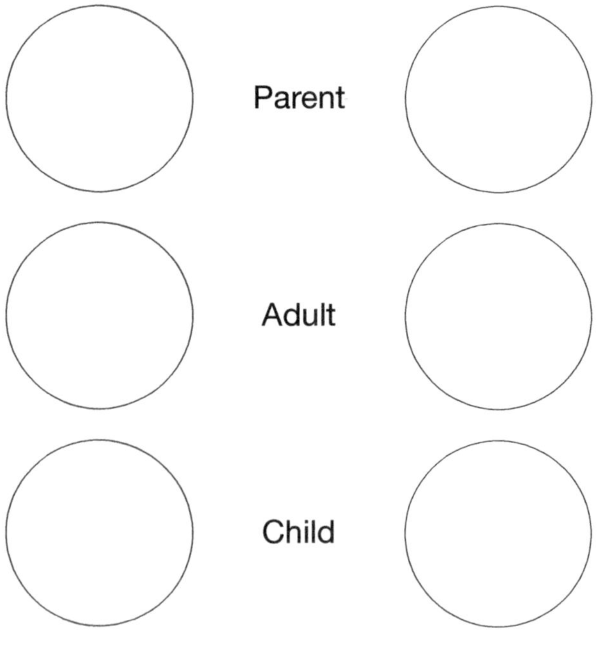

Figure 4.1. The Three Emotional Levels of Transactional Analysis.

In terms of transactional analysis, a labile, intoxicated, or personality-disordered patient may demonstrate child-level reactions to certain questions by personally attacking the clinician (just like in vignette #3 in the previous chapter and depicted in figure 4.2). The personal attack is an emotional reaction. Such reactions can be an actual avoidance of answering the question or reflection of the patient's mental state. Nevertheless, depending on the personal attack, the clinician can be distracted from the task if the clinician reacts versus responds to the patient's personal attack. The child-ego role that some patients and family members portray is discussed further in chapter 6 as part of a strategy to thwart power struggles.

Other than a patient's blatant refusal, a personal attack can be an attempt to gain some kind of emotional power in the exchange to avoid answering questions. The natural emotional reaction could intimidate the clinician and disrupt the interview. The clinician who is not mindful of the different emotional levels can react out of the misperception that the childish attack is a parental judgment on them (depicted in figure 4.3). The clinician who emotionally reacts likely does so in a personally defensive manner and so the interview gets off topic and instead of gathering patient information, it becomes about the clinician.

Furthermore, the personal attack is frequently stated in the language of a cognitive distortion such as an assumption, personalization, or emotional thinking. The assumption is typically mind reading or jumping to conclusions (You think that I am just going to say whatever you want me to say?). The personalization statement is blaming the clinician for feelings (You are pissing me off!). The emotional thinking is a demonstration of avoidance but

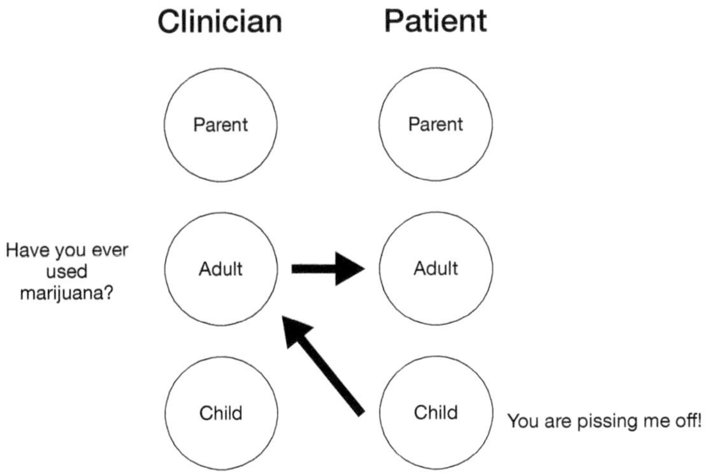

Figure 4.2. The Patient Responding from the Child Emotional State.

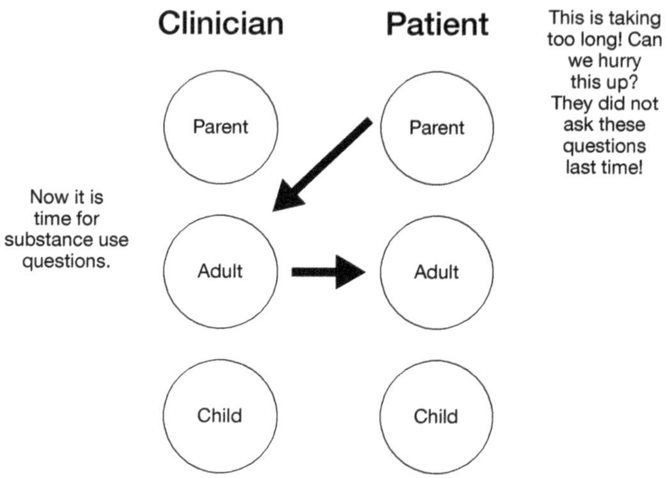

Figure 4.3. The Patient Responding from the Parent Emotional State.

does indicate some of the patient's mental status (I just feel that you are out to put me in the hospital against my will!). All these personal attacks are usually delivered by patients in a loud, angry tone that is the child level of emotion.

A challenge for the clinician is to avoid interpreting the patient's anger as being from the parental role and thus playing the child role. A person playing the child role assumes that the anger of another person means that you have automatically done something wrong and offended someone. It is as if you are an ignorant child doing or saying something that you should not have done; you "blew it," and the consequence is that you made another person mad. Given this, it is surprisingly natural to go to the child role since it is so emotional in nature.

Human beings are emotional creatures, and emotions such as anxiety and anger are essentially "radars" that impulsively prompt a person to act in immediate fashion to protect or defend one's self when there are insufficient facts that the other part of the brain can analyze. Part of the clinician's professional development and refinement is learning to operate in the factual, adult level of emotion to stay on task and gather clinical information.[7]

The clinician can stay in the adult level by practicing the clinical skill of a calm tone of voice at a normal speaking volume. The reality is that a calm tone of voice is initially an acting job where the clinician must stay in a rational frame of mind and practice *modified boredom*.[8] Methodically discussed in chapter 6, modified boredom is an unemotional tone at a normal if not lower volume and perhaps a slower pace. Modified boredom gives an impression that the clinician is emotionally in control and has emotional power in the situation.[9] The tone of modified boredom can return the interview back to the necessary formality to complete the task.

The clinician's use of modified boredom in the face of a patient's outbursts and non-compliance in an interview has two typical outcomes.[10] The first outcome is that the patient synchronizes emotionally with the clinician by calming down and returning to a manner of cooperation with the interview. The second outcome is that the patient continues to escalate in the child-emotional state, which is an illumination of the patient's pathology and emotional inability to continue participating in the interview.[11] The second outcome of using modified boredom is not as frequent as the first outcome.

In cases where the patient and a collateral source such as a family member are escalating by way of arguing, the clinician can use modified boredom in a directive fashion. The clinician can state to all parties in the interview that while this is a stressful situation, it is important to stay focused on this interview. However, it may be better that the clinician simply state that it is better if the rest of the interview is conducted by talking to one person at a time separately.[12]

In concluding this section, it serves to say that "modified boredom" can serve as an emotional stabilizing or equalizing force in most cases where the patient becomes escalated. The clinician practicing the modified bored tone of voice indeed can sound calm and in control when the patient is escalating. More times than not, the patient will calm down to match the clinician, but escalated patients with narcissistic traits and/or who are under the influence of alcohol and drugs may continue to escalate, elucidating that they are exhibiting a child level of emotional or ego functioning. As a clinician continues to practice the technique, the clinician indeed experiences more scenarios and actual confidence where the practice of modified boredom truly becomes the feeling and demonstration of being calm.

Compensating with Assertiveness

Modified boredom is a complement to assertiveness. Assertive language is not passive or aggressive language, but a style of direct communication for standing up for rights and needs. In the context of the assessment interview, assertiveness is the clinician's professional stance. With cooperative patients, the expression of assertiveness does not go beyond the level of normal human conversation because the patient is compliant and following basic directions. With challenging and non-compliant patients, the clinician must use assertiveness scripts in an intentional if not extraordinary fashion in the same modified bored tone of voice to demonstrate structure and order in the situation.

Assertiveness is also usually spoken in terms of scripts. The scripts usually start with "I." Most sentences are subject-verb-object where "I" is the subject. Some examples include the following:

- I need you to calm down.
- I regret to inform you, but that requires me to make a report to protective services.
- I cannot let you out without an assessment.
- I cannot do that.
- I would like for you to go sit down.
- I (or we) cannot have you act that way.
- I will need to conduct an assessment before you can be admitted.
- I cannot continue the assessment until you answer the questions.

The list can go on, but the clinician should avoid directive statements that start with the word "you." Such a sentence can be received as an aggressive statement that has a higher risk of escalating the situation.

How a clinician is received when assessing a patient accompanied by family members as a referee amid conflict is common with the child/adolescent population. In that context, effective and respectful communication with caregivers can be the difference between the caregivers being assets or liabilities. Chapter 7 focuses on using assertiveness and compassion as de-escalation skills to assist in maintaining a safe environment and accomplishing an assessment in emotionally escalated and volatile encounters with child/adolescent patients and their families.

Fortifying Modified Boredom and Assertiveness with Direct Eye Contact

The clinician's assertiveness and modified bored tone of voice must be fortified with consistent direct eye contact.[13] While direct eye contact can be considered rude in some cultures, in clinical settings, it makes the clinician present as attentive, empathetic, confident, and in control of the situation, and it can motivate patients to talk about difficult and sensitive issues.[14] Without it, the clinician looks shy, uninterested, uncaring, and as if they are not listening to the patient and collateral source.

Direct eye contact is not a staring contest. It involves breaks every few seconds to look at screens for typing or writing on the interview form or maybe even to look away briefly to survey if anything else is going on or even for thinking of responses. Most of the time, the clinician is looking at the face or gazing in the direction of the client's face so it appears that there is direct eye contact.

How much direct eye contact is necessary varies based on a patient's emotional state. A labile individual with low ego strength (whether child or adult) may present as overly sensitive, vulnerable, and defensive if they yell "Don't look at me!" However, a frustrated patient may indicate that they feel that they are not being heard by yelling, "Are you listening to me?" The first situation was the client telling the clinician there was too much eye contact while the second was saying that there was not enough.[15] While most patients will not seem to care, those situations are existential indicators about the patient's personality and emotional state and do not necessarily mean there is something wrong with the clinician's level of eye contact.

Softening the Possible Abruptness with Introductions and Transitions

Another subtle element in addition to eye contact is the clinician's use of introductions and transitions between interview sections. This compensating element goes back to the emotional reality that the interview questions are intrusive and seeking intimate information that in any other setting is none of the clinician's business. While the clinician has an authoritative clinical need for the information, asking the questions out of the blue can come across as rude and abrupt. The use of introductions and transitions gives the patient appropriate notice about the nature of the questions and the opportunity to get ready to give answers on sensitive subjects.

A common introduction that is helpful for the assessment interview goes by the AIDET acronym. It was pioneered by Quint Studer and stands for

- acknowledge
- introduce
- duration
- explanation, and
- thank you.

This is a way of providing humanity to patients who are in a vulnerable situation. The idea of saying "thank you" to a patient in such a stressful setting can be awkward, but it can be saved for the end to thank the patient and family for trusting thc clinician in sharing the personal information. Saying such a "thank you" at the end of the interview can enhance if not restore the dignity of a patient and their family given the potential demoralization of being vulnerable with the clinician and sharing their problems, traumas, and pain during a dark crisis. An example of how this might look could go something along the lines of the following:

> Welcome to Riverbank Hospital. My name is John, and I will be completing an evaluation with you. The evaluation should take between thirty to fifty minutes, at which point I will discuss your case with one of our psychiatrists or nurse practitioners. According to your demographic form, it seems you are here due to depression. While we will certainly address those matters in today's interview, there are several other topics we discuss with every patient. Keep in mind some of the questions I ask you may seem strange, bizarre, or not related to why you are here. Thank you for entrusting us with your care.

Meanwhile during the interview, transitions alert and help a patient emotionally prepare for sensitive questions by reducing the shock. A transition is a simple introductory cue to a section that can provide segues between different topics. They are particularly helpful for sensitive topic sections that include:

- Trauma and abuse
- Sexuality (depicted in vignette #2)
- Drug and alcohol use (depicted in vignette #1)
- Suicidality
- Psychosis

Even with transitional statements, severe reactions to these subjects cannot be prevented, and it is not the clinician's fault if a patient reacts in such a way. Furthermore, the use of transitions does not guarantee a patient will answer sensitive questions, but it lessens the likelihood that the average patient will demonstrate shock and resistance when asked.[16]

A person with below-average functioning due to intellectual disability, intoxication, psychosis, or personality disorder can obstruct if not intentionally sabotage their assessment despite the clinician's strong interviewing skills. The impacts of acuity and ability on a patient's potential to engage and participate are explored in chapter 5.

The Rules of Confidentiality

In connection with the matter of shock and transitions, the reality is that the assessment clinician is a mandatory reporter. While reporting laws vary from jurisdiction to jurisdiction, the clinician must report abuse and neglect and make duty-to-warn reports. The clinician should be oriented and updated as to what the current, local regulations are to stay in compliance. The clinician is challenged in this situation to balance legal requirements of confidentiality with the legal requirements of reporting abuse, neglect, and cases of a duty to warn.

Otherwise, confidentiality is tied to credibility and validity in such interviews. There is an inherent principle that patients will talk about their problems and trust professionals if there is a confidence that their information is kept private.

At times, a patient may make a disclosure that must be reported. A patient may admit that they have abused someone (specifically a child) or have thoughts of wanting to hurt or kill someone. Children may report that a parent has hit them or touched them in the interview. If the clinician tells the patient after the fact that they must report it, then it can be taken as an act of betrayal by the patient. The patient can then shut down or become disruptive for the duration of the interview.

Depending on the pathology of the patient and the family, they can instigate drama by complaining about the clinician for breaking confidentiality. In these cases, there is not a substantial leg for the complaint to stand on, but it can be disruptive to the interview and stressful for the clinician.

Given these situations, the clinician's best option is to make it a practice to state the rules of confidentiality at the beginning of every interview. A suggested script for such rules is as follows:

> This interview is confidential; however, there are two exceptions under state[17] law since I am a mandated reporter. If someone reports abuse or neglect, I may be required to make a report to the protective services. If someone reports that they want to hurt or kill someone, I am required to do a "duty to warn." Otherwise, what is said here will stay here.

Logically, this statement of the rules could provide a chilling effective for people to withhold some admissions of homicidal ideation and abuse. However, it also gives the clinician a leg to stand on when people report abuse, neglect, and homicidal ideation.

If the clinician has used the confidentiality script at the beginning of the interview and the patient still makes a disclosure, it is up to the clinician to decide whether they will tell the patient (and/or family/parent) that a report will be made.[18] Depending on how difficult or contentious the interview was, it can be appropriate to say nothing further to the patient and/or family to reduce the likelihood of further disruption in the interview setting.

Sometimes the patient may make the disclosure of homicidal ideation or abuse and then ask the clinician: "Are you going report what I said?" The clinician should be forthright and with a modified bored tone of voice say something along the lines: "I regret to inform you that I am required to report what you said." If the patient begins to escalate, it is an indicator of the patient's pathology or possible intoxication. If it is an emergency department, the clinician may need to step back and let the medical staff decide how to handle the situation. If the patient is escalating in the admitting department of the hospital, the clinician should consult with the supervisory personnel as to the best means to proceed with the patient's behavior. Otherwise, many patients will demonstrate acceptance of the clinician's answer and say nothing more.

CASE VIGNETTES

The following section consists of three vignettes demonstrating use of the different interview strategies and skills.

Vignette #1: The Patient Resistant to Answering Questions about Substance Use

The patient is a thirty-three-year-old female who presented to the hospital admitting department at about 5 pm on the day of assessment. She stated on her intake form that she came due to alcohol use, heroin use, and suicidal ideation. She had denied any use of alcohol today. She had already reported that she had thoughts of wanting to kill herself by overdosing on heroin.

Clinician: This question is about alcohol and substance use. Do you smoke or vape?

Patient: Yes.

Clinician: What age did you start?

Patient: About fifteen.

Clinician: How much do you average?

Patient: Whenever I can bum a cigarette.

Clinician: How much did you smoke in the last twenty-four hours?

Patient: I don't know . . . two cigarettes.

Clinician: When did you have your first drink?

Patient: About fifteen. Can we hurry this up? I don't remember all these questions the last time I was here.

Clinician: I am asking the questions that are in every interview. Now, when did you have your last drink?

Patient: Today at noon.

Clinician: Hmm. I am going to have to go and get the breathalyzer to see how much is in your system.

Patient: Do you have to? You are pissing me off!

Clinician: You are entitled to your feelings, but yes. I have to understand how much you have in your system so we give you appropriate treatment.

Patient: This is stupid s--t. You're really stupid! How the hell did you get your job? I want to talk to your supervisor.

Clinician: I cannot have you act like this, and the assessment cannot go on without your cooperation.

By following through with the breathalyzer, the clinician found out that the patient had a blood alcohol level of 0.16. The patient had withheld the information that she had consumed a half-pint (236 milliliters) of vodka in the hours prior to coming. For assessment purposes, she was intoxicated but evidenced a high tolerance of alcohol use and was either lying about her use or being a poor historian. The clinician resumed the interview.

Clinician: Now, how much have you been drinking per day?

Patient: I don't know.

Clinician: We need to know so you get appropriate detox treatment if you are drinking daily.

Patient: I get drunk every day on whatever is around.

The clinician continued with the interview at the same pace, and the irritated patient was avoidant in the rest of the interview. However, the patient cooperated with the questions about opiates and the detox scale questions. The patient evidenced a Clinical Institute Withdrawal Assessment score of six and a Clinical Opiate Withdrawal Scale of eight. She was admitted under mental health criteria because she said that she had been suicidal and her detox scores were not high enough to be admitted under substance use criteria.

This vignette demonstrates that many patients who come in with dual diagnosis complaints do not accurately and truthfully report what they are using and how much they are using. The patient's smoke screen of irritability and anger apparently masked that she was minimizing her alcohol use and that her substance use was a sensitive subject. By practicing modified boredom, assertiveness, and ignoring the patient's personal attack, the clinician was able to persevere through the patient's emotion and get relevant assessment information that had implications for appropriate treatment given that the patient reported getting drunk daily and was legally intoxicated at the time of the interview. In terms of transactional analysis, the patient was acting like a child and the clinician stayed in the adult role.

Vignette #2: Talking about Sexual History

The patient is a twenty-four-year-old male who was sent for assessment by his probation officer at the intensive outpatient program due to his testing positive in a random drug screen. The structured interview has questions about sexual history that are irrelevant to the patient's reason for presentation. This vignette demonstrates using the technique of transition.

Clinician: These questions are about sexual history. I prefer to tell people that this is none of my personal business because sexual matters are private, but the assessment has a section on it. Are you a male who was born a male?

Patient: Yes.

Clinician: How do you define your sexual orientation?

Patient: I'm straight.

Clinician: Do you consider yourself to be a sexually active person?

Patient: Yes.

Clinician: Do you have any issues or problems of a sexual nature?

Patient: No.

Clinician: Do you consider yourself to be practicing safe sex?

Patient: Yes.

Clinician: Have you ever engaged in sexual behavior that could be considered to be dangerous or risky?

Patient: Yeah.

Clinician: Can you share what the nature of that was?

Patient: I have had unprotected sex a few times.

Questions about sexual matters from a total stranger are intrusive and can be rude. The clinician softens the intrusiveness by affirming that it is a private matter and using the modified bored tone of voice. Affirming privacy and confidentiality in an emotionally neutral manner provides some sense of emotional boundary on multiple levels so that the patient provides a valid answer.

Vignette #3: The Arguing Family Members

The patient is a fifteen-year-old female brought in by her mother. The reasons for assessment on the intake form were: "suicidal, disobedient, out of control." In scanning the patient and her mother, the clinician noted that the mother and patient appeared to be tense and irritable. The clinician started out the assessment with the preamble.

Clinician: Hello, my name is David. I am an assessment clinician and I have been with the hospital fifteen years. This is a structured interview that will hopefully take about forty minutes depending on how much there is to discuss. The interview is confidential, but there are two exceptions under state laws. If someone reports abuse or neglect, I may have to call the protective services. Also, if someone reports that they want to hurt or kill someone, I have a duty to warn that person. So, what brought you today?

Mother: Well, my daughter has been running out of the house and hanging with a group of kids who have been doing drugs. She also has been . . .

Patient: STOP LYING MOM!

Mother: . . . running off and seeing this older guy who she has been sending inappropriate pictures to. She is always on her phone and when I asked for it, she said that she was going to kill herself.

Patient: THERE YOU GO AGAIN, JUST LYING MOM!

Mother: WELL, YOU ARE. I SAW THE PICTURES ON YOUR PHONE!

Patient: YOU HAVE NO RIGHT TO TAKE MY PHONE AND GET INTO MY PERSONAL BUSINESS!

Clinician: I think that this is only going to work if I talk to you separately. So, I am going to talk to your mom first. (Addressing the patient) I will come back to you. I definitely need to hear what you have to say, because I hear and see how upset you are. But for now, could I have you go back out to the waiting room? I will see you in a bit.

The clinician showed the patient back to the waiting room and interviewed the mother for the collateral information. The clinician went down the interview script looking for criteria that would indicate the need to hospitalize the patient.

Clinician: Now let's try this again. So, your daughter has been running from the house and hanging with a bad group. What else?

Mother: She has been on her phone constantly and she stays up all night on it and her grades have gone down.

Clinician: Have you heard her make any statements of her wanting to hurt herself, kill herself, or wanting to die?

Mother: She frequently says that she wants to die when she gets mad or when I demand that she put her phone up.

The mother showed the clinician a text message earlier today relayed by a friend of the patient that the patient stated she thought about killing herself.

Clinician: Today or yesterday has she made any statements of a way that she was going to kill herself?

Mother: I did not hear her say anything.

Clinician: Has she previously been admitted to a hospital before because she wanted to kill herself?

Mother: No.

Clinician: Has she ever engaged in self-harm? Deliberately cutting on herself?

Mother: I don't know.

Clinician: Has she made any statements of wanting to kill someone else or threatening to punch people?

Mother: No.

Clinician: Has she been hitting people or been physically aggressive in the home?

Mother: No.

Clinician: What is her sleep and appetite like?

Mother: She eats a lot of junk food, but she eats, and her sleep appears to be decreased. I suppose she is getting about five hours a night.

Clinician: Is she taking her showers, brushing her teeth, and changing her clothes on a daily basis?

Mother: Yeah, she does that. She is particular about her appearance.

The clinician then had the mother and patient trade places.

Clinician: Okay, now why did your mother bring you in here?

Patient: She demanded my phone. I told her that if she took my phone or turned off my phone, I would fight her and then I would kill myself.

Clinician: Let me jump in now with these questions: Have you had any thoughts of wanting to go to sleep and not wake up?

Patient: Yes.

Clinician: Have you had any thoughts of wanting to die or kill yourself?

Patient: No.

Clinician: Have you done anything, started to do something, or prepared to do something to end your life?

Patient: No.

The clinician asked the rest of the interview questions with the patient alone in the room. The patient denied suicidal ideation beyond wanting to go to sleep and not wake up. The patient last reported feeling that way a day ago. She denied homicidal ideation and psychosis and was oriented to reality. The patient denied being abused or neglected. She reported that she was having problems sleeping. The clinician staffed the case with the next psychiatrist on rotation, and the patient was referred to the hospital's partial hospitalization program as she did not meet criteria for inpatient.

The clinician used modified boredom and assertiveness to intervene immediately in the situation and keep the interview going with minimal to moderate disruption. The clinician was careful not to take sides in the argument; the clinician went with interviewing the parent alone first out of respect and because the patient was upset. The patient was calm enough by the time the clinician came back to her and cooperated with all the questions. The structured interview also was a stabilizing element in that the clinician sought to assess criteria for services (which is its purpose) and not why the patient and mother had conflict.

CONCLUDING THOUGHTS

The assessment interview is normally structured in a way that allows for reliability in ultimately determining whether a patient meets criteria for inpatient admission. It is intended to be an impersonal professional-patient encounter, but it can be an intensely emotional experience.

It is crucial to be mindful that the interview is not a normal event in the life of an average person and the patients are making themselves highly vulnerable in answering the questions. The patient is likely a willing participant but also naturally reluctant given the normal sense of embarrassment and defensiveness that comes with such personal disclosures. Given the natural emotion, it serves that a personality-disordered and/or intoxicated patient can show more intense and irrational reactions that include personally attacking the clinician out of their impaired cognitive state and lower ego functioning. In interviews with a patient and family members, arguments can break out over why they are there, which distract and impede the clinician from completing the interview. The skills and strategies the assessment clinician uses in this setting consist of rehearsed scripts as demonstrated in this chapter and the practice of emotional intelligence.

Emotional intelligence starts with an understanding that the clinician is compensating with formality and maintaining an adult level of emotion. The school of transactional analysis is a most helpful lens of understanding the dynamics and strategies by which the clinician thoughtfully responds and not impulsively reacts to the patient's emotional defensiveness that can come across as outbursts and personal attacks.

Outwardly, the clinician's response is calmness; it is not a natural emotional state but must intentionally be cultivated. This is a professional development challenge because humans naturally react emotionally in an escalating manner to perceived threats and challenges in everyday life. A way to develop and cultivate the calm adult state is by practicing modified boredom in both facial expression and tone of voice. For many, it is easier to think and sound bored than to think and sound calm. Modified boredom combined with assertiveness sends a message of stability in the average interview and emotional power when patients are escalating and can emotionally cue patients to de-escalate.

Besides the paraverbal cues of assertiveness and modified boredom, the clinician can keep the interview emotionally moving using introductions and transitions. Introductions and transitions can reduce emotional shock and re-install emotional boundaries between the patient and client and produce patient compliance with the interview.

In the end, a clinician should be mindful that patients being assessed do not want to be there. They do not want others to know that they are there. They do not feel good, and they would rather not answer the intrusive questions you are going to ask them about embarrassing subjects and regrets. The clinician frequently has the emotional challenge to conduct the assessment interview that must be addressed in rational ways.

NOTES

1. There may be some truth in the physical discomfort claims by detox patients.
2. At times, the same type of patient is not going to be cooperative with the physician either.
3. This is in accordance with the curve of ability.
4. The use of titles also establishes the roles in the professional-client relationship.
5. If the patient has a choice of a different title, the clinician should use it. Nonbinary individuals may eschew any title.
6. E. Berne, 1964, *Games People Play*, New York: Ballantine Books, 23–28.

7. It has been the opinion of the authors that many who have entered the helping professions and left were unable to achieve this emotional development. It is a form of emotional intelligence.

8. While not very intellectually sounding, it is a "Fake it until you make it" concept.

9. Sounding bored sends a subtle but powerful emotional message that the clinician is not scared or fearful of the situation. The clinician may still be internally nervous, and that is appropriate.

10. In cases of escalating patients, modified boredom can come across as a form of "gentle firmness."

11. A personality-disordered individual can play off the lack of emotional reaction by alleging that the clinician does not care because the clinician is not reacting emotionally. Such individuals may act in a confrontive/judgmental/bullying fashion toward the clinician and any other staff to intimidate and manipulate. In this situation, modified boredom can also be conceptualized as "ignoring" by not reacting to the patient's bullying behavior. The modified boredom approach can irritate the patient further because no one is joining them in the escalated state of emotion.

12. Such interviews are at risk of becoming family sessions, where the clinician is being triangled in Bowenian manner into a conflict which the clinician may or may not be trained to handle. Nevertheless, the argument distracts from the task at hand and extends the length of the interview. Furthermore, both the patient and collateral source may be hindered from disclosing important clinical material. Both parties should be redirected to focus or be separated if they continue to be escalated.

13. A. C. Berman and D. Chutka, 2016, "Assessing effective physician-patient communication skills: 'Are you listening to me, doc?'" *Korean Journal of Medical Education, 28*(2): 243–49.

14. J. K. Hietanen, 2018, "Affective eye contact: An integrative review," *Frontiers in Psychology, 9*: 1587.

15. Both situations are emblematic of individuals with personality disorders.

16. The curve of ability is applicable here. A labile person with personality disorder and possibly under the influence of substances is still likely to act out. A person with a personality disorder tends to lack the internal or ego strength to cope with simple emotional distresses that come with unpleasant topics and subjects. A reasonable person who is cognitively intact is likely going to cooperate.

17. *Province* or whatever applicable governmental district can be substituted in place of "state."

18. If a regular therapist is on the receiving end of a report of abuse or homicidal ideation, it is considered incumbent on the therapist to tell the patient to attempt to maintain or preserve a therapeutic relationship. Given that the assessment clinician does not have to develop the same level of therapeutic relationship, withholding disclosure that a report has to be made is not as crucial.

Chapter 5

Suicide Assessment

In its essence, suicidal ideation is a matter of life or death; someone is thinking to some degree about ending their life. Much of the suicide assessment material out there is more for outpatient therapists and healthcare providers about recognizing suicidality and suicidal risk in patients; however, suicide ideation is the center of the emergency and admission assessment. It is a prime reason for presentation and the primary liability of this work. Whereas it is important for the average mental health and medical professional to recognize when a patient is at risk for suicide and pose the important questions, the assessment clinician is going to ask directly whether the patient is suicidal in every interview.

As stated earlier in this book, the assessment clinician does not necessarily have to develop the therapeutic relationship to the extent that an outpatient therapist does with the client. The patient is in the assessment interview for a narrow purpose and will not have a multiple session encounter with the clinician. Therefore, the assessment clinician can be straightforward about suicide more so than the outpatient therapist and not necessarily worry that the patient will fail to return out of being offended. The assessment clinician is not excused from being respectful to the patient, but the expectation is that this interview will be conducted versus that a therapeutic relationship is formed.

Therefore, assessing suicidal ideation in this context should be straightforward with a few twists and turns. The assessment interview is a methodological approach to determine whether criteria is met and is not an act of shooting arrows in the dark. Most patients are willing to discuss their suicidal ideation, while some will play avoidance games with the clinician. Another twist is the existence of impulsivity, poor insight, and judgment where a patient can claim suicidality and then demand to leave; it suddenly does not seem to matter that they just said that they had a plan to kill themselves. The assessment clinician is often challenged to hold a straight course in conducting the interview, establishing criteria, and then rendering a treatment recommendation despite the twists, turns, and distractions.

The straight course that the clinician must maintain is based on criteria. Criteria are objective standards for admission to the hospital. The criteria are based on safety risk: immediate versus potential. The immediate risk criteria can vary based on the patient's intoxication or mental status. When the patient meets a criterion for immediate safety risk, the recommendation should be inpatient admission for the patient's safety. When the patient has a potential safety risk, other factors must be considered to determine whether the patient should be admitted as an inpatient. Learning the criteria should be an expected part of a clinician's job orientation and whenever it is changed by the managed care organizations.

Up front, the difficult reality is that not every "suicidal" patient will meet the criteria to be admitted because there are degrees of severity of suicidal ideation that can be divided into immediate safety risk and potential safety risk. The job of the clinician in this case is to be the eyes and ears of the hospital and the reviewing physician and be as thorough and objective as possible in ruling out whether criteria for immediate safety risk is met. The clinician should be able to articulate when a patient reporting suicidality is and is not meeting criteria for admission based on safety risk.

Compared to an outpatient therapist seeing a client in office and having a panoply of conversations in the context of a therapeutic relationship, the assessment clinician is having a structured dialogue with the patient that is going to specifically ask questions about suicide. The outpatient clinician bears the onus of screening for suicidality and its risk factors out of a wide variety of information, whereas the assessment clinician has one scripted dialogue with the patient solely for the purpose of answering the questions. Evidence-based practices and managed care organizations inform and dictate the script to yield information as to whether admission criteria are met. The clinician is still responsible for ensuring the interview is as thorough as possible to specifications. The new clinician is likely following the script with some trepidation but with experience confidence is gained in the act of suicide assessment.

There is some inherent fear in the matter of suicide assessment. While the liability factor is a chilling effect about suicidality, death also is frightening. Besides concern about life-damaging litigation and licensure board action, the clinician can bear the emotional weight that a patient could die because the clinician did not do a thorough job or effectively explain the situation to the psychiatrist. The clinician's best tools are conscientiousness and mindfulness.

However, there is some relief in that the assessment clinician is neither reinventing the wheel nor shooting arrows in the dark in evaluating suicide in the interview. The clinician is regularly the second or third in the chain of assessment when it comes to communicating with the patient about suicide. In emergency departments, the patient will have disclosed suicidality to nurses and physicians prior to the clinician being called in to conduct a more thorough assessment. The patient presenting to freestanding psychiatric hospital intake departments will frequently report on the intake forms that the reason for coming is suicidal ideation. Outpatient therapists and referral sources also may call the department prior to the patient's arrival with collateral information about what the patient has said and done necessitating assessment. Furthermore, patients will spontaneously disclose that they are suicidal when the clinician asks the usual opening question "What brought you here today?"[1] The clinician must follow the standard protocols to clarify the extent and severity of the patient's suicidality and produce normalized answers whether admission criteria is met.

The clinician can experience some stressful drama while trying to clarify whether the patient's suicidality is meeting criteria for admission; there can be a high degree of emotional conflict in the interview and process of assessment. Some patients will understate the level of suicidality. On the other hand, referral and collateral sources can overstate or exaggerate the level of suicidality. Family members may call after the fact and yell at clinicians answering the phone in admitting departments when a patient is not admitted. If a family member or significant other accompanies the patient into the interview, arguments can erupt that distract and lengthen the time to complete the assessment. The clinician is often challenged to negotiate this drama in a factual and rational manner, especially when it comes to the matter of suicidality.

This chapter focuses on the reality of suicide assessment in the emergency and admission interview. Most of the time, the criteria can be met by the report of the patient alone. However, there are other risk factors such as psychosis/delirium, substance use, and intoxication that must be considered when assessing a suicidal patient for possible admission. Collateral information from family and friends or other professionals can be compelling to admit a patient on an involuntarily basis, even when it contradicts what the patient reports. However, some of that information may not be factual or rational and must be clarified. Furthermore, it is an adjustment process for a clinician to ask patients about suicidality in a professional manner. Most of the time, suicide assessment is straightforward in this setting, but it is important for the clinician to be mindful of exceptional conditions.

THE CRITERIA OF SUICIDE ASSESSMENT: IMMEDIATE VERSUS POTENTIAL SAFETY RISK

In the hospital admission assessment, there is essentially a dichotomy: immediate safety risk versus potential safety risk. In the first category, the patient is obviously demonstrating suicidality that unmistakably suggests that if the patient is not made safe, the patient is a danger to themselves if they are not admitted. The second category says that there is potential danger but there are protective values and conditions that keep the patient resilient. If the patient lacks the protective factors, they could evolve to being a danger to self. This section follows the InterQual pattern for understanding the safety risk criteria.[2]

Immediate Safety Risks

Regarding suicidality, there are four essential categories of immediate safety risk. The patient attempted suicide. The patient is reporting suicidal ideation with a plan to do it. The patient may be reporting auditory (and maybe visual) hallucinations telling them to kill themselves. Furthermore, the patient may report that they are suicidal while intoxicated. All these clearly suggest that the patient needs to be admitted inpatient without question due to suicidality.

Command Hallucinations

Command hallucinations are a form of psychosis where the patient is reporting seeing things or hearing voices telling the patient to do something. Command hallucinations will more likely be auditory in nature telling the patient to harm self or others. The hallucinations can be unrelenting, and patients have been known to go and lie down in the middle of streets or pull an eye out because of the voices. A patient being interviewed will often volunteer at the beginning of the interview the experience of command hallucinations to harm themselves and the immediate recommendation is inpatient.

Did the Patient Make a Suicide Attempt?

The patient who has attempted suicide is recognized to have impaired insight and judgment and is disconnected from reality; they may still be desiring to end their life. They may also be having cognitive side effects and medical problems from whatever suicide method they used, especially overdosing.

The assessment clinician will typically encounter the patient who has attempted suicide in an emergency room or hospital room. A suicide attempt is intended to be a fatal injury and the patient will likely be on a seventy-two-hour psychiatric hold. By the time the clinician is called for assessment, the patient will be medically cleared and stable to ensure that they are safe to be moved to a psychiatric inpatient unit.

If the interview is not in an emergency department and the patient reports just having attempted suicide by ingestion of poison or overdose, the clinician should immediately stop the interview and consult a physician. In such conditions, the patient who claims to have ingested poison or an overdose should be taken immediately to a hospital by emergency medical services for medical clearance and possible treatment.

Many times, the patient will report a less lethal type of suicide attempt. Some common patient reports include the following:

- They tried to hang themselves.
- They put a gun to their head.
- They went to a bridge and almost followed through with jumping off.
- They laid down in the middle of a street.
- They tried to run out in traffic to get hit by a car.
- They tried to swallow some pills but then spit them up or threw them up.

Patients may report some bizarre suicide attempts, and in the strange situations it is incumbent on the clinician to staff with the doctor about the credibility of the patient's claim.

Regardless of the patient's report, in the end, *what matters is the patient's intent*. No matter how convoluted the patient's report, it is within their mental state that they had made the decision to act.

Is the Patient Reporting Suicidal Ideation with a Plan within the Past Forty-Eight Hours?

The patient who is thinking of a "plan" is contemplating a way or method of suicide. The patient may spontaneously report that they have been thinking of a "plan," which will make the clinician's job easier. Otherwise, the clinician will typically ask a progression of questions that include:

- Have you been having any thoughts of wanting to go to sleep and not wake up or wanting to die?
- Have you been thinking of a way you would kill yourself?
- (If yes) *How* have you been thinking of killing yourself?

An example of this progression is the Columbia Suicide Severity Rating Scale[3] that has been a multi-party collaborative effort that provides a sense of the extent of a patient's risk.

The suicide plan can be an existential matter. Related to the earlier list, some frequently stated plans include

- overdosing on pills,
- getting a gun and shooting themselves,
- hanging,
- jumping off a bridge,
- running out into traffic,
- cutting their own wrists or neck,
- wrecking their car by driving off the road or into a barrier or into oncoming traffic, or
- drowning self in a tub.

Sometimes the plan can be involved like electrocution or "suicide by cop," where a patient plans (or maybe even tries) to do something to get a law enforcement officer/peace officer to shoot them. The patient may come up with a bizarre plan that can go beyond the clinician's wildest imagination or what can even be stated here. In the end, what matters is that the patient reports thoughts of wanting to kill themselves by a specific method.

Time is a factor as to when a person reported the suicidal thoughts with a plan. There is a time window of the patient's plan, and that is between forty-eight and seventy-two hours. The essential view is that the patient is still within that window of vulnerability of acting on the thoughts of suicide.

While this discussion has been based on the InterQual outline, one more standard can be used in assessment: plan and intent. Does the patient state that they have a plan? There are manipulative individuals who will say that they have thought of all kinds of plans, but they may or may not have intention to do any of them.[4] The Columbia Scale questions provide the method to clarify whether the patient is going to follow through with the action. However, it can be expected that if a person is thinking of a plan for suicide, they are thinking of following through with it.

Is the Patient Suicidal and Intoxicated?

An intoxicated patient tends to be a more impulsive person and is at higher risk of acting on suicidal thoughts. Drugs and alcohol affect the brain and thus distort their thoughts and judgment.[5] Therefore, an intoxicated person reporting suicidal ideation even without a plan is an immediate safety risk. The intoxicated person may not be reporting a plan for suicide or a suicide attempt, but given the propensity for impaired judgment, the recommendation should be inpatient hospitalization.

Potential Safety Risk

When it comes to potential safety risk, if it is established in the interview that the patient reported having suicidal thinking but denied having a plan or intent, then clinician can make a *rule out* for safety question by asking: "Do you believe that you would be safe if you were not admitted to the hospital tonight?" (This is discussed in vignette #4.) A patient unable to contract will not readily say yes or they might immediately say "no." If the person is unable to "contract" for safety, then the recommendation should be for inpatient admission.[6]

If they say that they are going to be okay, then it is incumbent to consider potential risk. Potential risk is on a case-by-case basis, and it has more to do with children than it does with adults. The child or adolescent may have behaviors that are dangerous, and the caretaker or parental figure may not be able to maintain (in their opinion) safety.

Where you go next in the case of a potential safety risk is the impairment in the patient's functioning. Is it severe, moderate, or mild? How disrupted is the patient's life due to the depression or anxiety that is part of the symptomology at the time of the assessment? There is a distinct possibility that the patient may still meet criteria for coming into the hospital if they are unable to function in any part of their life to include their activities of daily living (hygiene, going to work, eating, changing clothes).

Self-harm is a quandary to discuss as part of a potential safety risk. There are two different schools of thought: the European school of thought of self-injurious behavior and then the North American school of thought of non-suicidal self-injury. With non-suicidal self-injury, a person engages in self-injury without actual intent to die but to express emotional pain, seek attention, belong with a crowd, experience endorphins, or feel something to break the numbness.[7] Self-injurious behavior, on the other hand, views self-harm occurring in the presence of suicidality. Regardless of the view, many people who engage in self-harm may be suicidal at the time of the interview. What is crucial when a patient reports self-harm is that the clinician clarifies that it is not for the intent of suicide.

The quandary of potential safety risk due to suicidality can always be clarified by staffing with the on-call psychiatrist or the next psychiatrist on rotation. Sometimes patients reporting suicidal thinking and other symptoms will be "on the line" between needing inpatient admission and a referral to a partial hospitalization program. Decisions about where a patient should go should be deferred to a psychiatrist.

APPLYING THE CURVE OF ABILITY

The curve of ability was discussed in chapter 3, and its application to suicide assessment pertains to whether the patient demonstrates the capability of answering questions in a valid manner. The patient in the "High Acuity/Low Ability" quadrant (IV) demonstrates little to no ability to answer the questions due to their psychosis, intoxication, or medical condition. The inability to answer the question should be considered an immediate safety risk. A comatose person or a person who does not wake up should be sent off for immediate medical clearance; this person may have overdosed or is in medical crisis. However, a patient who is wide awake but demonstrating severe psychosis to the degree of inability to answer questions about suicidality should be considered an immediate safety risk because they are unable to answer whether they are having suicidal ideations. The psychotic patient in this quadrant also is not able to consent to treatment. The patient fitting in this quadrant should be involuntarily admitted if they do not need medical clearance.

The patient in the "High Acuity/High Ability" quadrant (III) is expected to be straightforward in answering about their suicidal ideation with some exceptions. Typically, most high utilizers, who frequently come for admission, say exactly what is necessary to present as an immediate safety risk. However, a high utilizer with narcissistic or anti-social personality traits may be treatment-savvy, gamey, and give puzzling, limited, or vague answers as to the extent of their suicidal ideation. This type of high utilizer presents as

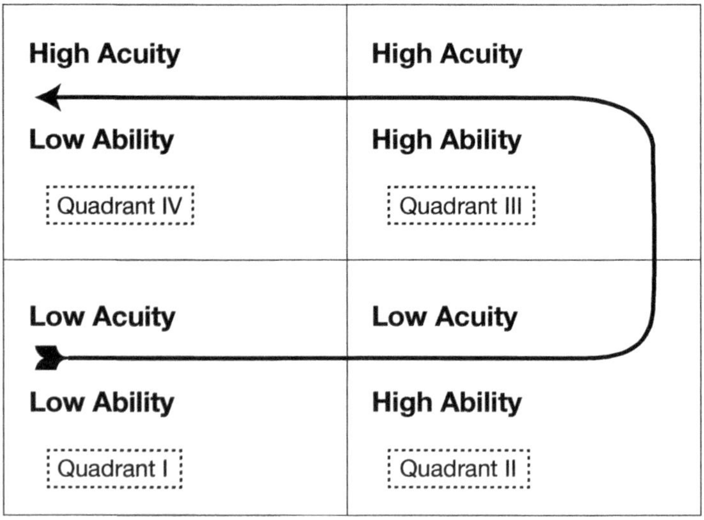

Figure 5.1. The Curve of Ability.

dancing between the higher two quadrants in that they are suicidal but refuse to participate any further in the interview. Any attempts to get the narcissist or anti-social to elaborate are often met with what amounts to be verbal abuse of the clinician and the patient being disruptive. Barring personality disorder traits, a person of normal intelligence who would present as otherwise well-adjusted and mature will give a direct yes or no answer to questions about suicide.

The patient in the "Low Acuity/High Ability" quadrant (II) will report as having suicidal ideation in the potential risk category. They will likely just have thoughts of suicide, but they are not meeting the criteria to be admitted. They are likely reporting the feelings of hopelessness and helplessness, and any thoughts of suicidal ideation are without a plan or intent. They will likely be fine with a referral to the intensive outpatient or partial hospital programs versus being unable to contract for safety.

The patient in the "Low Acuity/Low Ability" quadrant (I) may or may not be able to say whether they are suicidal due to intellectual ability or being non-verbal. This type of patient will likely be brought by a caretaker for assessment for unsafe behaviors and may not comprehend most of the questions. Most if not all of the interview will depend on the collateral source for descriptions of the behavior patterns.

THE VALUE OF COLLATERAL SOURCES

In general, collateral information is gathered about a patient from others who know the patient outside the hospital in the home or community or who have witnessed the suicidal comments or behaviors. Collateral information can be of great value as it provides crucial details that the patient is either unable or unwilling to talk about. Given what symptoms are, patients may

- be resistant to treatment,
- be non-compliant with the interview out of anger (such as an adolescent),
- have poor insight and judgment about their symptoms, or
- be unable to talk due to the influence of drugs or alcohol.

Sometimes there is a combination of conditions such as a drunk and angry individual who is refusing to cooperate with the interview. A collateral source can give the necessary factual information that is crucial to making a patient safe.

Collateral information can come before, during, or after the interview. The referral source such as a therapist, physician, or employer may call in advance. The patient may have a family member, friend, or acquaintance present in the interview. However, the patient may not want anyone else in the interview and have one or more people with them in the waiting room, and the clinician should ask them if they have anything to report. Much of the information depends on the dynamic or relationship between the patient and the collateral source.

However, there are caveats about using collateral sources. Such sources may have agendas and distort reality. While there is some logic to have a loved one or family member present in the assessment, it is an unusual, awkward, and distressing experience, and so the collateral source's language could be emotional. However, dysfunctional family dynamics and a collateral's personal psychopathology can mean a report that is a distortion of the reality. The person accompanying the patient or calling in to the office may be emotional and non-factual by using superlatives and making statements that are cognitive distortions.[8] The cognitive distortions include mind reading (projection), generalization, magnification, and catastrophizing. Examples of these non-factual reports include the following:

- They are having suicidal thoughts.
- They are very suicidal.
- They said they are suicidal.
- They are "really" suicidal.
- They are extremely suicidal.

At a minimum, these reports amount to be the opinion of the collateral source and not the facts of the situation, the patient's statements, or even the patient's behaviors.

There is a potential here that the collateral source may be dysfunctional or toxic and providing a skewed picture of reality. They may wield emotional power over a patient to get an assessment out of the collateral source's own personal issues. Some collateral sources may have personal agendas to punish or control a patient by making claims that are not true but they are stated in a factual manner. However, some collateral sources just do not have insight as to their own lack of emotional intelligence and inability to distinguish facts and feelings. While the clinician cannot be a mind reader as to the intentions and motivations of such collateral sources, the challenge is to sift out the facts.

What makes the sifting tricky is that the collateral source may be escalated and yelling at the clinician in an angry tone of voice while sitting beside the patient in the interview. The clinician can be intimidated by the collateral source.[9] The collateral source may themselves be treatment savvy or talking to the clinician as they do to other family members. This emotion amounts to an embellishment that can distort reality. Again, while the clinician cannot be a mind reader, the clinician needs to sift through the emotion and get to the facts.

There are some techniques the clinician can use in getting to the facts. When a collateral source is calling prior to the interview, the clinician can ask pointed, clarifying questions. If the collateral source engages in the mind reading that says "They are suicidal," the clinician can ask:

- What exactly are they doing or saying that tells you they are suicidal?
- When did they do this?

If the collateral source says "They're really suicidal," the clinician can ask questions such as:

- What exactly did they do?
- What exactly did they say?
- When did they say this to you?[10]

If the collateral source is being overtly emotional and disruptive to the order of the interview,[11] which hinders the patient's talking, the clinician should talk with the patient alone by taking them out of the room away from the collateral source or redirecting the collateral source to leave the room. A way to say this is in a "bored" tone of voice to the collateral source in the room, "I think I had better talk to you both separately. Can I have you step outside for a few minutes? I will call you back in, and I will talk with you alone, separately."

Much of the time, the collateral source will comply with the request. If the collateral source is escalated themselves and refuses to comply, then the clinician may have to seek the assistance of security, other staff, or emergency room personnel to coax or persuade them to leave the room.[12]

BECOMING ACCUSTOMED TO ASKING PATIENTS ABOUT SUICIDE

Asking patients about suicide tends initially to be awkward. It is a very personal question that potentially is intrusive and offensive.[13] Also, to disclose that one is suicidal is a naturally shocking matter that would be a crisis for the patient, but also to those around them. However, the nature of the interview gives the clinician license because the assessment is not an everyday discussion in the life of an average person. The clinician is one of those professionals formally delivering a service for specific purposes.

Given the formality, the clinician's attitude and tone should be respectful and calm. Since "calm" is often hard to achieve, a helpful alternative, which will be expanded on in chapter 6, is "modified boredom." The bored tone is an intentionally unemotional tone of normal, conversational volume, which can assist in keeping the overall emotional level of the assessment down. It should be expected that the average patient coming for assessment is making themselves vulnerable in disclosing the suicidality, and the unemotional tone helps provide a sense of professionalism and non-judgmentalism; this is an everyday occurrence for the professional who knows how to handle it. With time and experience, the new assessment clinician naturally develops a professional style in responding to the suicidal patient.

VIGNETTES OF SUICIDE ASSESSMENT

Vignette #1: A Straightforward Situation

A thirty-four-year-old female presented alone for assessment. She had written on both of the intake forms: "Thoughts of wanting to die." The following was the interview.

Clinician: What brings you here today?

Patient: I've been having depression, and I was thinking about killing myself today.

Clinician: What kind of thoughts have you been having?

Patient: I was thinking about taking a bunch of pills to end my life.

Clinician: When did you last think about doing that?

Patient: I thought about it all day.

At this point in the interview, it has been established that the patient is evidencing an immediate safety risk due to the suicidal ideation with a plan within the past forty-eight hours. The clinician will still need to finish the interview and might have to repeat some of the suicide assessment questions that the patient just answered, but the patient should be admitted to the hospital for safety.

Vignette #2: A Family Argument

A twenty-eight-year-old male is accompanied by his mother into the interview. The reasons given on the intake forms are depression and anxiety. The patient responded to the opening question that he had been depressed lately and that his mother thought he needed to come in and talk to someone. The clinician then asked his mother about her point of view. His mother repeated that the patient had been depressed. A family argument erupted when the clinician specifically asked the patient about suicidal ideation.

Clinician: In the past twenty-four hours, have you had any thoughts about wanting to go to sleep and not wake up or thoughts of wanting to die?

Patient: No.

Clinician: Have you had any thoughts of killing yourself?

Patient: No.

Mother: Come on, Billy. You said earlier today that you were thinking about cutting your wrists and taking some pills because you just wanted to end it all.

Patient: Shut up, Mom! Why did you have to open your trap and blurt out my business?

Clinician: Ma'am, when did Billy last say that?

Mom: Around noon today.

Clinician: Mr. Billy, your mother reported that you were having thoughts of cutting your wrists to kill yourself. Any comments on that?

Patient: No . . . and Mom, you need to shut the f— up.

It is noted that the patient did not deny the mother's collateral report and the remainder of the interview was tense and the obviously angry patient was resistant to talking. The patient and mother traded a few more verbal jabs, but the clinician was able to get through the interview. The clinician later pulled the patient out of the room to ask the interview questions about abuse and sexuality. At the end of the interview, the clinician discussed with the patient and mother that the patient was meeting criteria for inpatient admission.

Vignette #3: The Personality-Disordered Patient Who Wants to Leave

A thirty-four-year-old female presented to the admitting department and spontaneously told the clinician in the hallway in a strangely calm voice that she had wanted to kill herself by jumping off a bridge. The clinician had the patient complete the intake paperwork and met with the patient in about fifteen minutes. During the interview, the patient became irritable and argumentative in answering the questions.

Clinician: These are the questions about suicide. In the last seventy-two hours, have you had any thoughts about going to sleep and not wake up or thoughts about wanting to die?

Patient: No.

Clinician: You mentioned earlier to me in the hallway that you had thoughts of killing yourself by jumping off a bridge. Have you been having any other thoughts of killing yourself?

Patient: No. Can I leave? I don't want to stay in the hospital!

Clinician: You told me in the hallway that you had wanted to kill yourself by jumping off a bridge.

Patient: Oh.

The clinician's polite and minimal confrontation worked to get the patient off the topic of wanting to leave; the patient reluctantly completed the interview, and the clinician staffed the interview with the recommendation for inpatient. However, when the clinician came back to talk with the patient about the doctor's identity and the reserved bed, the patient again became argumentative.

Patient: I want to leave. I don't want to stay in this f-----g place.

Clinician: Here is the problem. You said that you had wanted to kill yourself by jumping off of a bridge. There is a choice. You can either sign yourself in as a voluntary patient or I will have to have you placed on a seventy-two-hour hold. Which one will it be?

The patient did not answer but sat down in response to the clinician's use of the "illusion of choice" intervention. When the registration clerk came, the patient refused to sign the admission paperwork. The clinician called the psychiatrist back and received an order to place the patient on a seventy-two-hour hold.

Vignettes #2 and #3 illustrate that some patients who are suicidal also have poor insight and judgment due to depression, personality disorder traits, or even substance use. They might conceal that they are having suicidal thoughts. They can also make explicit reports of being suicidal with a plan but then demonstrate the expectation that they should not face the natural consequences; this is often the poor connection to reality that comes with mental health issues. While there is the temptation to analyze the underlying conditions and reasons, an assessment clinician is best focusing on the basic facts and following through with the admission protocols in such cases.

Vignette #4: The Gamey Patient (Maybe I Am Suicidal)

A thirty-eight-year-old male for a "telehealth" assessment initially presented for gastrointestinal issues that were evaluated. The patient was experiencing homelessness and was recognized as a high utilizer to this emergency room. When he met with the physician's assistant to talk about the results just prior to what was supposed to be discharge, the patient then said that he was suicidal.

With the patient's claim of being suicidal, a referral for assessment was made and the clinician met with the patient via a teleconferencing platform. The nurse giving "report" to the clinician related the details.

Initially, the patient said he had several bad days, he was depressed, and he was not feeling well. He said nothing about being suicidal. The clinician then asked the set of questions about suicide.

Clinician: Are you having any thoughts of wanting to go to sleep and not wake up?

Patient: I'm not sure.

Clinician: Are you having any thoughts of wanting to die or kill yourself?

Patient: I think so.

Clinician: Have you done anything, started to do something, or prepared to do something to end your life?

Patient: I suppose so.

Clinician: What can you tell me about the suicidal thoughts that you have been having?

Patient: I have just been having suicidal thoughts lately given how bad things have been.

Clinician: How often do you have these thoughts?

Patient: I have them a lot.

Clinician: Have long have you been having them?

Patient: A long time?

Clinician: How many days?

Patient: Oh, I've been having them for years?

Clinician: Have you been thinking of a way that you would kill yourself?

Patient: I can think of a lot of ways I can kill myself . . . getting a gun, running out into traffic, jumping off of a bridge?

Clinician: But have you *actually* thought about doing one of those in the past two days?

Patient: Maybe.

The clinician went on with the rest of the assessment. The patient reported feeling hopeless, helpless, and lacking energy. Being homeless was a challenge to the patient being able to perform activities of daily living. The patient denied having homicidal ideation and all forms of psychosis. The patient reported smoking marijuana and drinking a thirty-two-ounce beer daily. At face value, the patient was not meeting criteria for inpatient, but he was not answering the questions clearly.

Being mindful that the reason for the assessment was the patient's initial report of suicidal ideation, the clinician took one more shot at clarifying whether the patient was meeting criteria for admission.

Clinician: If you were not admitted and instead referred to an intensive outpatient program starting tomorrow, do you believe you would be safe and not a danger to yourself?

Patient: No.

While it took a long time, and despite the vagueness of the gamey patient's answers, the clinician had established that the patient was meeting criteria for admission because of the inability to contract for safety.

Part of the initiation of the assessment clinician is the gamey patient who avoids clear answers about suicidal ideation. There are numerous reasons this kind of patient plays games, but it tends to be related to personality disorders. In this case, there is often a thinly veiled agenda of malingering, but the master's level assessment clinician should not be acting as a judge; all clinical recommendations should be officially made by a psychiatrist. Regardless of the reason, such patient behavior is frustrating to establish whether criteria are met for inpatient admission. The very human clinician can personally risk losing composure to a situation that is naturally frustrating.

Vignette #5: Another Gamey Patient: "I'm Suicidal and I Am Not Saying Any More"

A thirty-one-year-old female presented for assessment. The patient had a reputation of being a high utilizer and disruptive in the admitting department waiting area on a regular basis. She immediately demanded food when she came in and then quickly minimally and sloppily filled out the intake forms—"Suicidal! Voices!" After she ate, she covered herself with a blanket and yelled at the clinician when told that it was time for the assessment:

Patient: I'M SUICIDAL, AND THAT'S ALL YOU NEED TO KNOW!

Clinician: We still need to do the assessment. Please come with me.

The patient screamed as if she was annoyed and inconvenienced but did get up and go to the assessment room. The patient continued to demonstrate annoyance but allowed the clinician to take her vitals. She covered her head again but was at least sitting. The clinician attempted to proceed with the official interview script.

Clinician: What happened that you needed to come in?

Patient: I TOLD YOU! I'M SUICIDAL, AND THAT'S ALL YOU NEED TO KNOW!

Clinician: You wrote that you were hearing voices. What can you tell me about that?

Patient: I DON'T WANT TO TALK ABOUT IT!

Clinician: What is your living situation?

Patient: IT'S NONE OF YOUR BUSINESS!

Clinician: Look, these are the interview questions that are part of every assessment. It's nothing personal.

Patient: I DON'T CARE! I'M SUICIDAL. I'M HEARING VOICES, AND THAT'S ALL YOU NEED TO KNOW.

Clinician: Have you been drinking alcohol or using drugs?

Patient: IT'S NONE OF YOUR BUSINESS. I'VE BEEN HERE BEFORE LOOK AT THE RECORD!

The patient then left the room and went back and laid on the floor of the admitting waiting room and was laying on the floor in a fetal position while covered up by a blanket.

The clinician first talked with the supervisor who was familiar with the patient. The clinician then called the previous psychiatrist and reported the patient's behavior and statements. The psychiatrist accepted the patient for admission to the hospital.

This was anti-social behavior, and the patient had learned that she could manipulate the system by saying the bare minimum, refusing to cooperate, and then intimidating the admitting department staff. This patient looked like they fit in quadrant IV of the curve of ability. This manipulation can escalate to the point of disruptive or physically aggressively behavior to shorten the wait and speed up going to the unit. Depending on the hospital policy, the clinicians and other staff are stuck trying to maintain the peace in the waiting room in consideration of the other patients waiting for their assessments or for admissions. The kind of patient who typically engages in these behaviors is a high utilizer and becomes well-known to hospital staff, especially the clinician who can become familiar with the patient's behavior.

When admitted, this type of patient tends to be disruptive and not treatment focused. They tend to be verbally aggressive toward staff and other patients. Hospital administrations may eventually restrict the patient from future admission or prescribe protocols to clear the patient rapidly from the department.

Vignette #6: The Psychotic Patient Who Will Not Answer the Question

From time to time, the clinician will encounter a psychotic patient who is cognitively unable to participate in an interview. The patient may be behaviorally agitated and restless; they cannot sit still and will not respond to prompts to fill out forms and come into the room to be interviewed. Such a patient may be intensely pacing in the hall and will stop for nothing. The other option is that the patient is not answering questions or giving irrelevant answers to the questions.

The following is an example of a patient who is behaviorally cooperative but cognitively incapable. The patient's intake form was not completed despite it having been given to the patient upon entry two hours prior to the interview. The form had a name but had unintelligible scribbles on it.

Clinician: My name is David. I am an assessment clinician. I am going to do your interview. What happened that you came here for assessment?

Patient: *(The patient stares at the clinician for ten seconds.)*

Clinician: John, why did you come into the hospital to talk to us?

Patient: The hamburgers ran away.

Clinician: The hamburgers ran away? Where did they run to?

Patient: The water is purple. The floors and grass.

Clinician: John, are you having any thoughts of wanting to die or kill yourself?

Patient: The president of the United States.

After several minutes of this conversation, it was evident that the patient fit within quadrant IV of the curve of ability. The patient was psychotic to the point where he could not answer questions about being suicidal. Furthermore, it could be concluded that the patient had impaired insight and judgment to the point that the patient was unable to keep himself safe. The patient also could not legitimately consent to treatment. The clinician should consult the emergency department physician or the psychiatrist to obtain an order for involuntary admission for the patient.

Vignette #7: A Case Not Meeting Criteria for Admission

Just because someone reports having suicidal thoughts does not mean they must go into the hospital. This oversimplified scenario demonstrates use of the Columbia Suicidal Scale questions.

Clinician: What brings you in today for assessment?

Patient: I have been feeling depressed, and I cannot focus on my work. My sleep has declined, and I just do not feel like doing anything.

Clinician: Have you been having any thoughts of wanting to go to sleep and not wake up?

Patient: Yes.

Clinician: Have you had any thoughts of wanting to kill yourself?

Patient: No.

Clinician: Have you done anything? Started to do anything? Or prepared to do anything to end your life?

Patient: No.

The clinician went on to some questions that elaborate on suicidal ideation.

Clinician: So, what can you tell me about the thoughts of suicide you have been having?

Patient: I have just been thinking about dying lately. I have been feeling hopeless and that people might be better without me.

Clinician: Have you *actually* thought about ways that you might die or kill yourself?

Patient: No. I have children who need me.

The clinician proceeded with the remainder of the interview and learned that the patient had been having problems with sleep and appetite and that some activities of daily living have slipped. The patient was able to go to work, but they were having concentration issues there. The patient denied homicidal ideation and psychosis. At the end of the assessment, the clinician summed up the information of the interview and asked a clarifying question.

Clinician: As I have understood your situation today, you are having symptoms of depression where you have had some thoughts of wanting to go to sleep and not wake up but not to kill yourself. You have had some problems with sleep and appetite, and it is harder to do your normal activities. If we were to recommend you to go to an intensive outpatient program where you could be seen tomorrow and not admit you to the hospital, do you believe that you would be safe?

Patient: Yes.

Clinician: Okay. We will go in that direction.

The patient in this case readily said that they were safe. A patient stopping and showing hesitation should be reconsidered for admission. However, again in this case, this patient said without hesitation that they were okay with the plan to admit to an intensive outpatient program.

CONCLUDING THOUGHTS

Suicide assessment is essentially the center of the admission interview and is part of the script. Unlike the outpatient therapist, the assessment clinician will directly ask the patient the necessary questions to establish whether the patient meets criteria to be admitted. The criteria for admission are typically evidenced based and ordained by insurance or sub-contracting managed care organizations and organizations accordingly craft structured interview scripts.

The clinician does not have to worry about offending the patient by asking questions about suicidal ideation. The professional should not be shocked when a patient is reporting being suicidal but should maintain a calm tone of voice that can be achieved by practicing a modified boredom and taking the emotion out of possible responses. The clinician should care within the limits of the encounter but also focus on the task of completing the interview.

The patient is expected to be able to give clear answers as to whether they are psychotic. However, psychosis/delirium, substance use, and intoxication must be considered when assessing a suicidal patient for possible admission. Not all patients are capable and/or forthright in answering the questions, and with some consideration, collateral information from family, friends, and professional service providers in the community can be helpful in establishing whether criteria for admission is met based on suicidal ideation.

Through the lens of the curve of ability, the refusal or inability to answer questions about suicidal ideation should be considered the same as an immediate safety risk in most cases. The exceptions are children and adolescents with lower intellectual functioning who are brought in due to physical aggression or out of control behavior that meets other criteria for inpatient admission. It is conceded that there are high utilizers (as demonstrated in vignette #5) who appear to exploit this condition, but it is ethically preferable to err on the side of caution when it comes to suicidality.

Going back to the human aspect, the new assessment clinician can expect to feel nervous in asking for the first time if a patient is suicidal. Furthermore, there is some healthy fear over the reality of suicidal ideation and behavior. With practice, the conscientious clinician can confidently and effectively assess patients for suicidal ideation.

NOTES

1. The patient will essentially be asked more than once if they are suicidal. The first time is an open-ended question and the following questions are closed ended.

2. This outline is based on structure of the "InterQual" criteria (2013) McKesson Corporation. InterQual is one of several industry standards. InterQual was sold to Change Healthcare. It is an evidenced based system of utilization management.

3. K. Posner, G. K. Brown, B. Stanley, D. A. Brent, K. V. Yershova, M. A. Oquendo, G. W. Currier, G. A. Melvin, L. Greenhill, S. Shen, and J. Mann, 2011, "The Columbia–suicide severity rating scale: Initial validity and internal consistency findings from three multisite studies with adolescents and adults," *American Journal of Psychiatry, 168*: 1266–77.

4. The matter of borderline personality disorder comes into play here where a "borderline" is chronically suicidal and suicide is an answer to solve their problems. The dynamic of the interview in these cases is that the borderline is highly emotional and may or may not be testing the interviewer or pushing emotional limits with the interviewer with emotionality such as sarcasm, rage, or near-panic. The patient can also challenge the interviewer by personal attacks as to the interviewer's competence or perceived apathy ("You are a jerk" or "You don't really care about me"). It can challenge the clinician to stay calm and rational during the interview.

5. R. Hufford, 2001, "Alcohol and suicidal behavior," *Clinical Psychology Review, 21*: 797–811. See also C. J. Cherpitel, G. L. Borges, and H. C. Wilcox, 2004, "Acute alcohol use and suicidal behavior: A review of the literature," *Alcohol Clinical and Experimental Research* (5 Suppl): 18S–28S.

6. Many agencies eschew the use of the terms "safety contract" or "contract for safety" in documentation when a person is suicidal. It invites a liability risk.

7. A. Steinhoff, D. Ribeaud, S. Kupferschmid, N. Raible-Destan, B. B. Quednow, U. Hepp, M. Eisner, and L. Shanahan, 2021, "Self-injury from early adolescence to early adulthood: Age-related course, recurrence, and services use in males and females from the community," *European Child & Adolescent Psychiatry, 30*: 937–51.

8. A. T. Beck, 1976, *Cognitive therapy and the emotional disorders*, New York: International Universities Press. Typically, the concept of cognitive distortions is used in psychotherapy to encourage depressed and anxious individuals to change their thinking from emotional patterns to rational and factual patterns. However, emotional patterns can emanate in the way people communicate to others. Feelings are not facts, and a collateral source could be communicating their personal feelings and not the facts of the patient's statements and behaviors.

9. A collateral source like this tends to have had practice in being intimidating to a wide variety of people and can personally attack the clinician by engaging in insinuation and name-calling, and demanding to talk to someone in management.

10. If a clinician is taking a phone call from a collateral/referral source in advance of the patient's arrival, these questions are also applicable. Writing down explicit details makes it simpler for a colleague who eventually does the interview.

11. The collateral source and patient can start arguing and attempting to triangle the clinician in as a rescuer or as a therapist in terms of Bowenian therapy.

12. An irate and paranoid parent may not cooperate with such a request. The lack of cooperation by the collateral should be documented and reported to a supervisor in case the collateral makes a complaint or grievance.

13. Most patients are not going to come across as defensive or claim they are offended by this question. A patient who would come across as stating they are offended is one with a personality disorder.

Chapter 6

The Disruptive, Aggressive, and Anti-Social Patient

People who get into the helping professions intellectually assert that they want to help others with their problems. However, the reality of patient anger is one of those baptisms by fire or professional rites of passage, because, while logically, it is an expression of unmet need and pain, the stress of being on the receiving end of it may make a clinician re-evaluate why they wanted to be in this profession.

People get mad for various reasons. Some of them are valid, and some of them at face value are ridiculous, but at times "anger" is danger without the "d" on the front of it. People who are angry can be loud, threatening, and impulsive to the point of being physically aggressive. While we would like to be wrong, the fine print of working as an assessment clinician is that there will be experiences (or at least the risk) of patient scenarios like these:

- A patient punched the door of the assessment clinician's office yelling, "What the hell is going here? If I'm not taken to the unit in five minutes I am going off!"
- A patient screamed, "if you don't unlock that door and let me out of here, I will break it down and walk out myself!" The patient then threatened to call their lawyer.
- A patient grabbed a clinician in the hall and said, "The bitch who evaluated me lied about what I said and is trying to force me into admission. That is illegal, and my dad is a judge. I think you better let me go as well as have her fired."
- A man in the waiting area detoxing from heroin yelled at another, "STOP LOOKING AT MY WOMAN!" He then went across the room and hit another patient waiting for assessment.

The assessment clinician will encounter angry patients. The patients may be mad out of a sense of vulnerability and defensiveness because their egos are hurt for having to come and be assessed. The anger may be related to the eroding effect that depression or mania has on the ability to tolerate the environment. The patient may be under the influence of substances or detoxing from them. The patient may also be expressing unmet needs. Regardless of triggers, there is an increased likelihood that the angry patient will be uncooperative with the interview or exhibit some degree of disruptive and aggressive behavior.

The clinician may be the one who must step in to intervene. Sometimes, the intervention can be simple as meeting physical needs. However, there are safety risks associated with disruptive, aggressive, and/or anti-social patients. The risks are enhanced when the patient is intoxicated, off their medication, and has a trauma history. Angry people are also vulnerable people and thus can irrationally attack the clinician and others in the assessment area in addition to damaging or destroying property.

This chapter discusses a variety of strategies for clinicians to manage and de-escalate situations with angry and aggressive patients. There are concrete safety measures that include taking transponder devices where available and maintaining increased personal space from the patient. In more touch-and-go situations, the clinician may have to speed through selected questions to establish whether criteria for admission is met. This chapter further discusses the concept of modified boredom and introduces an option we call *paradoxical affirmation of emotion* which are both verbal de-escalation strategies.

ANGER DUE TO UNMET HUMAN NEEDS

The curiosity about those scenarios at the beginning of chapter is "Why did they do that?" Without more information, it is tempting to judge that "The guy's a jerk" or "The person is an idiot," but that is only a luxury that the bystander can enjoy. On the other hand, the clinician must quickly identify what triggered the behavior and either safely calm the person down or call for help to intervene. The trigger to an individual's anger may be ascertained by simply asking the person, "What's the problem?" At other times, the clinician may need to consider what is bothering them using Abraham Maslow's Hierarchy of Needs (1943).

Maslow suggested human beings are motivated to meet needs and the drive to meet them grows stronger the longer they are unmet. Maslow's Hierarchy of Needs tiers are illustrated here, with the first needs being the most basic and necessary for survival and the last related to growth as a human.

1. Physiological needs (e.g., air, water, food, shelter, sleep, clothing, reproduction)
2. Safety needs (e.g., personal security, employment, resources, health, property)
3. Love and belonging (e.g., friendship, intimacy, family, sense of connection)
4. Esteem (e.g., respect, self-esteem, status, recognition, strength, freedom)
5. Self-actualization (e.g., desire to become the most that one can be)[1]

Hence, a patient who has been without food and water may act out in anger order to meet their needs.

A patient's needs should be considered when you observe them to be angry, disruptive, or aggressive. Can you apply Maslow's Hierarchy of Needs to the previous situations to hypothesize what the individuals are trying to accomplish. That is, the purpose of their behavior is to achieve what? Even if a person is identified as having an unfulfilled "esteem need," it cannot be overlooked that they may also have unmet basic needs for food, water, dry clothing, and a sense of safety. Also, clinicians should be mindful that some patients may be off their medication and/or experiencing drug or alcohol withdrawal which would be deficiencies in "safety needs."

The acting out due to unmet needs ranges from passive aggressive comments to escalated behavior that includes

- yelling,
- insulting others/making verbally aggressive comments,
- threatening to act out,
- slamming or kicking doors,
- hitting walls or property,
- throwing chairs or other available objects, and
- attempting to assault or actually assaulting another person (clinician/other patient/bystander).

These are all safety risks and hence the clinician's priority is to ensure the safety of others who are present (family members, guests, patients, colleagues, and self). Thus, understanding the reasons for patient behavior can mean quicker and smoother de-escalation and risk reduction. The initial confrontation of inappropriate behavior always carries some risk that the escalated patient may attempt to

- intimidate the clinician or other staff with verbal threats and encroachment,
- instigate other patients,

- engage in property destruction, or
- assault the clinician or other individuals.

However, these potential threats can be minimized through behavioristic psychoeducation such as this material and practicing role-plays of such clinical situations with colleagues or classmates.

What is the purpose of behavior? From a behaviorist perspective, a person may act inappropriately

- to get attention,
- to get access to an item/activity, or
- to avoid something.

Can you match the reasons with the scenarios described at the beginning of the chapter? The first scenario is someone wanting access to an item/activity (in this case going to the unit). The second scenario is someone trying to avoid an activity (in this case admission to the hospital). The third situation is someone expressing anger by seeking attention and instigating milieu problems (if I am going to be miserable, then you are going to be miserable). Here are some other scenarios where the purpose of the behavior must be assessed (what they are trying to achieve) to deescalate effectively.

Joseph

Joseph is an adult patient who had been waiting for two hours for assessment and had yet to be interviewed. The waiting room was full of other patients who also had been complaining about the wait time, and it appeared to have rubbed on him. Joseph got upset and kicked over his chair in the waiting room yelling, "I guess they just evaluate the patients they want to see!"

Joseph's primary goal was to *gain access to an activity*, which in this case was to get assessed. He may have gotten a secondary gain of attention. Again, assessing what the patient or guest is upset about allows for proper intervention in terms of how to redirect them.

Telling an angry patient simply to "Calm down" or "Stop yelling" may set a limit but it will not address the root cause of the behaviors and may further escalate emotion.[2] On the other hand, explaining to Joseph the volume of people being evaluated, giving him concrete information with respect to when he will be seen, and providing him with options will likely be more effective in helping him calm down.

Mary

Mary is an adult who presented seeking inpatient detox. However, she did not meet criteria to get admitted. She was offered an intensive outpatient referral.

She became upset, demanded to be admitted, and started ripping papers off the walls. She threatened to call her therapist who referred her to the hospital and said, "She WILL get me admitted!"

The purpose of Mary's threat to call her therapist was to create a power struggle and ultimately to *gain access to an activity*. Knowing she is seeking inpatient treatment explains her acting out and provides direction for dialogue such as asking,

- Is there some reason you are opposed to the outpatient program?
- Do you know what the outpatient program offers?
- Would you like to know your options for potential admission for detox?

Again, the context explains the origin of Mary's behavior and offers the opportunity for direct dialogue to resolve the problem instead of again just telling someone to "Calm down."

Timmy

Timmy is an eleven-year-old boy who was assessed due to aggressive behavior at school and threatening to harm his younger sister. The recommendation was that Timmy be admitted but he needed a COVID-19 swab. Timmy refused the COVID-19 swab, ran from the assessment room, and barricaded himself behind some waiting room chairs. He was clearly demonstrating avoidance.

Hopefully, Timmy will comply if the clinician talks with him in a respectful manner. This includes the clinician stating (in a tone of modified boredom),

- an understanding of why Timmy is hiding,
- giving him information on the procedure, and
- offering some sort of incentive that will hopefully result in compliance with the test.

Simply pulling him out from the chairs and forcing the nose swab could cause undue physical and emotional harm for Timmy and any involved staff, which we will discuss further in the next section.

Jackie

Jackie is a twenty-nine-year-old female who presented to the hospital in what appeared to be a manic-like state with grandiose delusions/delusions of grandeur and homicidal ideation. She was inconsistent in her psychosocial information. Jackie said that she wanted to be admitted inpatient because she did not feel safe. Her previous psychiatrist accepted her for admission.

While waiting to go to the unit, Jackie announced that she did not want to stay. She told a different clinician in the department that the clinician who did her assessment was a "liar." She then denied that she ever said anything about hurting herself or others. Jackie said that it was another patient in the waiting room who told her to say what she said in the assessment. She then threatened to sue the hospital and to hurt the other patient in the waiting room.

The purposes of this anti-social-like behavior appear to be discrediting the hospital and its employees as well as to intimidate other patients. Understanding what Jackie is trying to accomplish can negate power struggles, and simply separating her from other patients may minimize or eliminate the risk of aggression.[3] All of this should create a situation of minimal risk and harm.

However, the caveat when attempting to engage in discussion is that agitated patients who are in an active state of florid psychosis, under the influence of alcohol or another substance, detoxing from alcohol or opioids, or a combination of all of these can be highly impulsive and incapable of engaging in dialogue to determine the purpose of behavior. Part of the impulsivity includes being unable to regulate emotion. There is periodically no time for analysis or verbal intervention because some patients escalate impulsively to a level of therapeutic crisis and physical aggression. At the point of physical aggression, it becomes a matter of restraining the patient by whatever safety or crisis intervention method/system/technology the hospital subscribes. The clinician comes into situations at different levels of emotional volatility on the part of the patient making the analysis of antecedents impossible.

Ironically, some patients initially capable of talking become escalated even during attempting to dialogue and negotiate with them. Somewhat akin to the curve of ability discussed in chapters 3 and 5, they are incapable of coping with the problem and escalate in frustration or rage. There are risks that must be considered when attempting to talk with agitated patients.

RISKS ASSOCIATED WITH THE DISRUPTIVE, AGGRESSIVE, AND/OR ANTI-SOCIAL PATIENT

The disruptive, aggressive, and/or anti-social patient is a threat to the safety and well-being of the clinician conducting the assessment both during and after the interview. The disruptive patient can intentionally interfere with the clinician's keeping the interview on track. This not only compromises the validity of the assessment but potentially leads to interruption, argument, and aggression from the patient. If the situation were to escalate to physical aggression, there is imminent risk of the therapist and/or patient being injured.

But is there any way we can predict if a patient will act violently? How does a hospital enhance its risk management to minimize injury for said violent behavior? According to previous research in the mental health community, "A history of violence has been consistently shown to be the best single predictor of future violent behavior."[4] Consequently, it is critical a clinician know as much as possible about the client they are going to interview.

A patient's history of violent behavior or lack thereof can be ascertained through intake of the individual; collaborative information obtained from family, friends, or providers; as well as by reviewing available medical records, if applicable. Furthermore, healthcare systems have trended toward instituting "flags" in the electronic medical record for patients with a history of aggressive or violent incident for future notification.[5] In addition to a client's history, a clinician can also examine presenting risk factors.

Risk factors that can alert the clinician to potential violence can include

- intoxication,
- acute psychosis (i.e., hallucinations, delusions, paranoia),
- symptom presentation (e.g., irritable, or angry affect, poor insight, judgment, or impulse control),
- history of child abuse, and
- medication non-compliance.

"Numerous studies have shown that having been a victim of child abuse or having grown up in a violent home increases a patient's risk of violence later in life."[6] Other risk factors for escalation and aggression include an unwanted, involuntary admission and another patient instigating a fight in the hospital waiting room. A patient who becomes disruptive, argumentative, or hostile post assessment either in a waiting room, hallway, or at the clinician office door also presents a risk of potentially harming the therapist, other patients, guests, or themselves, not to mention any property that is destroyed in the department as illustrated from the following sequence of events adapted from a real case situation.

Safety of the Therapist

Patient "John Doe" presented for depression and substance abuse. He reported suicidal ideation with a plan to overdose on pills. After the usual provider staffing, it was recommended that he be admitted to inpatient. However, he said that he wanted to leave. The clinician called the psychiatrist back and the doctor ordered a seventy-two-hour hold. The clinician took the patient into an assessment room and explained the doctor's order to be admitted involuntarily to the hospital. Mr. Doe started yelling and then shoved the clinician to the wall and attempted to tackle the clinician to the floor.

Safety of the Patient

The therapist attempted to put Mr. Doe in a crisis management hold. Both Mr. Doe and the clinician fell to the floor, and on the way down Mr. Doe hit his head on the corner of the desk. Mr. Doe sustained a laceration to the head. Other staff, seeing the incident on the video monitoring system, called a code, and the code team managed Mr. Doe and escorted him to the unit. Mr. Doe struggled during the management and further strained his shoulder and sprained a finger. In the process, several of the code team were exposed to possible blood-borne pathogens from Mr. Doe's head laceration.

Safety of Other Patients and Guests

Ms. "Jane Doe," who also came to be assessed, was sitting in the waiting room and became upset that her husband was physically managed and taken to the unit. She reacted with anger and confronted another patient who had appeared to be staring at her. She yelled, "What the hell are you looking at?" The other patient replied, "Nothing worth my time, psycho!" Ms. Doe got out of her chair, grabbed the other patient's hair, and pulled her out of her seat. Ms. Doe and the other patient were on their feet pulling and pushing on each other. A third person got up and attempted to break up the fight but got punched in the mouth. Staff eventually noticed the event and called another crisis code; security and the code team broke up the skirmish. Ms. Doe and the other patient sustained scratches and hair loss, and the intended good Samaritan got a cut lip.

Property Destruction

After her husband's restraint and the fight with the other patient, Ms. Doe continued to be escalated, and she engaged in property destruction. She turned over a recliner in the waiting room, which broke its arm. She then started kicking the department's exit door with her steel-toed boots. Furthermore, she tore down the mounted security mirror on the wall and threw it to the ground, cracking it. Security personnel put her into a crisis management hold, ending the episode. During the incident, Ms. Doe had caused hundreds of dollars of damage.

SAFETY MEASURES TO PROTECT THERAPISTS, PATIENTS, AND GUESTS

The discussed scenario leads to some questions. How do we as professionals intervene and minimize potential injury of patients, guests, staff, and ourselves? How do we manage these scenarios? What proactive strategies can we utilize to keep people safe? The following are some suggested answers.

- Ask security personnel to sit outside your evaluation office.
- Bring a transponder or alert device into the assessment.
- Position your desk near the exit of the evaluation office prior to the interview.
- Inform colleagues when you will be starting an assessment.
- If your facility has a camera system, inform the camera room to watch your office.
- Practice modified boredom in which you demonstrate the appearance of calmness no matter the circumstance.
- Provide your patient with options where applicable.
- Practice a good listening and "attending," allowing the patient the opportunity to express themselves.
- Practice rational detachment and do not take a patient's anger personally.[7]

When a patient is agitated, it may be helpful to accelerate the pace of the interview. While normally it is appropriate to conduct an evaluation slowly, asking follow-up questions, probing, pausing, and repeat-backs or paraphrases, in the context of a hostile individual it would be advantageous to speed up the pace. Another option in this context is to shorten the evaluation by only asking the essential questions to establish whether criteria are met for admission. In essence, the therapist would be first inquiring whether the patient has been experiencing the main criteria to establish whether there is an immediate safety risk. The main criteria include the following:

- Suicidal ideation with or without a plan
- Homicidal ideation with a clearly identified target and/or specific plan
- Withdrawal symptoms or history warranting detox admission (see chapter 8)
- Symptoms of severe psychosis

Once those four subjects are broached, the clinician can move onto mental status, substance use, psychosocial, and medical topics, in no particular order. The more agitated a patient is, the more likely they will be resistant toward discussing trauma and substance use history in total. The assessment is unlikely to be thorough, but with the agitated patient, it is sufficient to substantiate the necessary criteria to make a clear treatment recommendation.

Another option to expedite the assessment (when the agency or hospital uses computers) is to use a paper version of the interview. This allows the clinician to take information quickly and move rapidly between sections.

There is a likelihood that the assessment clinician working for a psychiatric hospital will receive some level of training in crisis intervention as part of job orientation. The crisis intervention training used by hospitals is a proprietary system that covers a spectrum of skills from communication strategies, therapeutic holds, and maybe up to marshal restraints. Not all outpatient mental health agencies subscribe to crisis intervention systems, and clinicians conducting emergency assessments for such organizations may benefit from additional study in crisis intervention and de-escalation,[8] but it is expected that an emergency room or other field setting such as a school has its own protocols for dealing with patient aggression.

The assessment clinician dealing with the aggressive patient must make a judgment call as to whether it is safe to conduct an interview in the first place. When possible, maintaining extra space between the clinician and the agitated patient can provide a sense of safety and boundary, whereas proximity can be received as intrusive and threatening. However, if a patient is being physically aggressive in some manner (hitting and attacking), it is too dangerous to interview the patient in that moment; that is rage, and the patient is not in a rational state of mind to cooperate and give appropriate answers. Unless the clinician has been trained and is competent to perform physical restraints within the organization's approved system, the clinician should defer physical intervention of an enraged patient to those who are trained. If a patient has escalated to the point of being restrained due to physical aggression, that precludes the interview and typically is grounds for inpatient admission.

Modified Boredom

If the patient has not reached a state of rage, there is some probability that the patient can de-escalate through the clinician's verbal and paraverbal skills to include active listening and empathy. The suggested strategy that was first mentioned in chapters 3 and 5 and being elaborated in detail here is "modified boredom."

Modified boredom is an internal script where the clinician tells or cues themselves to sound and look bored. It consciously requires the clinician to self-monitor. Modified boredom includes

- an unemotional facial demeanor,
- a bored but conversational tone of voice,

- a slower pace of speech,
- a lower volume, between normal conversation and above a whisper,
- slowing down the interaction by taking at least a few seconds before responding,
- intentional or deliberate moments of silence, and
- normal eye contact with the patient.

Inwardly, the act of modified boredom is a form of mindfulness in the crisis situation, but outwardly it looks and sounds calm to the patient. Dynamically, as discussed in chapter 4, it is the adult level of communication within the theoretical framework of transactional analysis that may cue the other person to match the same presentation which will equal de-escalation.

The internal script of modified boredom is more practical and realistic than a clinician trying to tell themselves to be calm. While initially it feels like a façade, it achieves the look of being calm and composed, which, again, can have a de-escalating effect on the agitated patient. Furthermore, the difference between regular boredom and modified boredom is that the clinician is actively listening and demonstrating empathy, whereas boredom infers disinterest and apathy.

By itself, modified boredom should be looked at as a vehicle by which to attempt negotiation and problem solving with the angry patient so that the matter is resolved or the patient is sufficiently de-escalated and that order is restored. The word "attempt" is often more applicable to the scenarios of patients making demands, especially when the matter is non-negotiable such as demanding to leave when they have been put on involuntary holds or wanting to go to the unit immediately.

Paradoxical Affirmation of Emotion

When the angry and escalated patient seeks something that is non-negotiable or is verbally making a personal attack on another person (such as another staff member or the clinician themselves), another de-escalation strategy is acknowledging the anger using modified boredom and giving affirmation or approval to feel anger. This can have a paradoxical effect per Erickson's theoretical framework.[9]

As illustrated in figure 6.1, interactions between two people that either lead to arguments or to physical aggression have a cyclical nature to them. Both participants contribute to the cycle of escalation by merely increasing the speed and intensity of their emotion and responses until it reaches screaming and/or physical acting out.

From the "dual process" perspective of thought processes, it can be viewed that both participants in an escalated exchange are thinking emotionally and

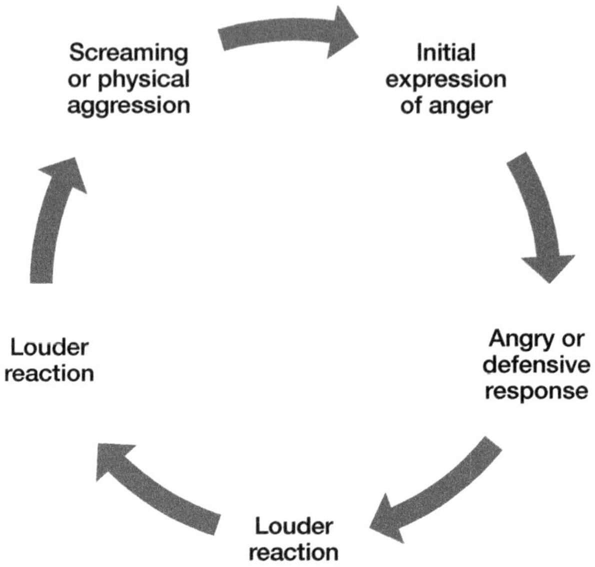

Figure 6.1. Cycle of Escalation.

thus impulsively. Bernstein calls this emotional thinking "fast thinking," as opposed to rational thinking which he calls "slow thinking."[10]

The escalated patient in complaining will likely either make a threat and/or claim to be a victim of the staff or other person (maybe a family member) whom they are personally attacking. The natural response is that of defensiveness, which can lead to a cycle of escalation between the two or more individuals. The emotional response is often intended to pacify or explain the situation, but it only adds emotional fuel to the escalation. The escalating, emotional patient is not thinking in a rational process and is unable to appreciate and accept the explanation and thus de-escalate.

Furthermore, the escalated patient may claim to be a victim at some level with a claim of being offended or unjustly treated to a third person, which has the potential of instigating a triangle of drama (discussed in a different context in chapter 11).[11] Depending on the response or reaction of the third person being triangulated into the conflict, the emotional escalation can then involve three or more people. The clinician using paradoxical affirmation can be the one being verbally attacked or the one whom the escalated patient is attempting to triangulate into the conflict with a third person.

Phrases that are examples of paradoxical affirmation include the following:

1. You can be mad.
2. You can be mad about this.

3. I can see that your mad about this.
4. I am okay with you being mad.
5. I am okay with you being mad with me.
6. It's normal to be mad in situations like this.

As illustrated in figure 6.2, by using these phrases the clinician is not joining the escalated patient in the emotional thinking but is disrupting a potential cycle or an existing cycle and is in a sense transcending the emotion of the situation by outwardly recognizing it.

Based on the experience of the authors, the two likely exceptions to the paradoxical affirmation working as intended include a patient who is grossly psychotic or under the influence of drugs and alcohol. The grossly psychotic individual may have internal stimuli triggering emotion that has nothing to do with the situation. The heavily intoxicated patient may have an impaired mental status and impaired cognitive processes to the point of being unable to engage in sufficient self-regulation to de-escalate. A savvy high utilizer with a history of "successful manipulation" through escalation and aggression also may fail to respond as hoped to the paradoxical affirmation.

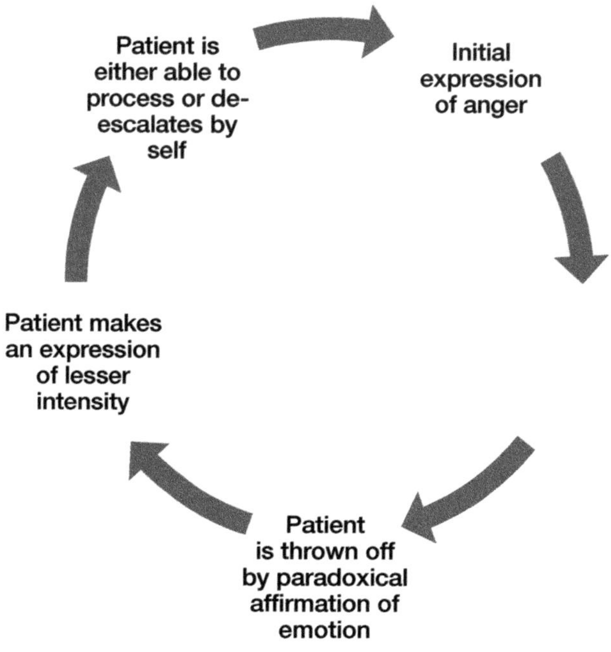

Figure 6.2. Disruption of Cycle.

CONCLUDING THOUGHTS

This chapter covered a variety of strategies for clinicians to manage interactions with angry and aggressive patients. While there are concrete safety measures, the clinician may have to do mini-assessments to establish the basics as to whether criteria for admission was met. The clinician can utilize the strategies of modified boredom and paradoxical affirmation of emotion that can cue a patient to de-escalate. When a patient is floridly psychotic or under the influence of alcohol or drugs, the safety measures and de-escalation strategies are of limited utility. It is reasonable to say that not every angry and aggressive patient will de-escalate in accordance with the recommended techniques and strategies; there will be restraints, seclusions, and (in emergency departments) the administration of sedation.

Anger is an emotion that has the connotation of impulsive and automatic behavior. Anger makes an individual louder and more impulsive in both speech and behavior. Conversely, the demonstration of anger in its aggressive and escalated forms does get the attention of others in the vicinity, and in the typical experience it elicits automatic reactions of fear or defensiveness. Humans tend to make automatic assessments of whether they are in danger and cringe or duck regardless. As human beings, clinicians also are going to react in automatic ways, but they are looked to as the authorities to intervene with the angry patient for the safety of others in a rational and methodical manner.

Not all clinicians will become specialists in intervening with disruptive, angry, or aggressive patients. Some clinicians will have more aptitude than others in such interventions. Nevertheless, being able to redirect an angry patient to focus and cooperate with the interview is a necessary skill whether it is an adult, adolescent, or a child patient.

The beginning clinician hopefully can observe seasoned clinicians deal with angry patients as part of job orientation. While this chapter has prescribed some techniques and methods that hopefully can be translated into action, the skill of dealing with angry patients is learned more by real-time modeling.

Even with following the model of a seasoned clinician, one hump to get over is dealing with being the target of a personal attack by an angry patient; the clinician must work internally not to take such attacks personally and practice some level of ignoring. Scenarios like one mentioned at the beginning of the chapter (*A patient grabbed a clinician in the hall and said, "The bitch who evaluated me lied about what I said and is trying to force me into admission"*) are surprisingly common. Many patients will come in and claim to be suicidal with a specific plan and then renege on their claim and demand to leave. They will get put on involuntary holds and with their poor insight and judgment start to blame the clinician in potentially vicious and abusive ways. Some of these patients can become school playground bullies in the way they persist in picking on clinicians and threaten them.

One last thought in dealing with angry and aggressive people. It is crucial to try and preserve the dignity of the patient, even if they are personally attacking the clinician like in the previous paragraph. Anger is a response to pain, and inherently the person exhibiting it is also indicating some level of vulnerability. An exception to this may be the high utilizer (discussed further in chapter 13) who, out of experience, repetitively acts out to circumvent waiting in the admitting department and escalating being taken to the unit. However, intervening with angry and aggressive people is an inherently therapeutic activity and how they are dealt with may contribute to or undermine treatment progress. To that point, inherently as discussed in chapter 5, modified boredom seeks to put forth an adult tone of voice and not a condescending tone to subtly show a patient basic respect.

NOTES

1. A. H. Maslow, 1943, "A theory of human motivation," *Psychological Review, 50*(4): 430–37.

2. With respect to limit-setting, "The therapist clearly points out the behavior that is unacceptable and maladaptive and explains why it is not acceptable. The clinician then explains the consequences if the behavior continues." For example, "Your yelling vulgarity at other visitors and tearing down our security mirror is inappropriate as we do not tolerate intimidation or property destruction here. If you cannot discontinue these actions, security will be called and you will either be physically managed or removed from the property." D. E. McNiel, 1998, "Empirically based clinical evaluation and management of the potentially violent patient," in P. M. Kleespies (ed.), *Emergencies in mental health practice: Evaluation and management*, 95–116, New York: Guilford Press.

3. This is clearly better than dividing staff against itself or involving other patients for a problem they did not create.

4. J. Monahan, 1981, *The clinical prediction of violent behavior*, Rockville, MD: National Institute of Mental Health; D. E. McNiel, R. L. Binder, and T. K. Greenfield, 1988, "Predictors of violence in civilly committed acute psychiatric patients," *American Journal of Psychiatry, 145*: 965–70; D. E. McNiel, 1998, "Empirically based clinical evaluation and management of the potentially violent patient," in P. M. Kleespies (ed.), *Emergencies in mental health practice: Evaluation and management*, 95–116, New York: Guilford Press.

5. D. E. McNiel, 1998, "Empirically based clinical evaluation and management of the potentially violent patient," in P. M. Kleespies (ed.), *Emergencies in mental health practice: Evaluation and management*, 95–116, New York: Guilford Press.

6. D. E. McNiel, 1998, "Empirically based clinical evaluation and management of the potentially violent patient," in P. M. Kleespies (ed.), *Emergencies in mental health practice: Evaluation and management*, 95–116, New York: Guilford Press.

7. The strategy is in essence the clinician practicing rational self-talk. Suggested examples of this are: *I am not responsible for the anger of others—I am only responsible for my feelings. I did not make this patient angry. This patient happens to have issues that contribute to their problems with anger. Anger is a sign that they are having problems coping with life and especially this situation. People with anger management problems are quick to blame others for their anger and slow to take responsibility for it.*

8. One worth mentioning is Gilliland and James' Model of Crisis Intervention that proposes a six-step strategy to manage individuals who are acting erratically. B. E. Gilliland and R. K. James, 2016, *Crisis intervention strategies*, eighth edition, Boston: Cengage Learning.

9. J. Haley, 1973, *Uncommon therapy: The psychiatric techniques of Milton H. Erickson, M.D.*, Oxford, UK: W. W. Norton. This cycle is also similar to the domestic violence cycle of L. Walker, 1979, *The battered woman*, New York: Harper & Row.

10. A. J. Bernstein, 2013, *Emotional vampires at work: Dealing with bosses and coworkers who drain you dry*, New York: McGraw Hill Education. This is a popular book that explains dual-process theory.

11. S. B. Karpman, 2014, *A game free life. The definitive book on the drama triangle and compassion triangle by the originator and author. The new transactional analysis of intimacy, openness, and happiness*, San Francisco: Drama Triangle Publications.

Chapter 7

Assessing Children and Adolescents

Variety may be the spice of life; however, that may not be so for the assessment clinician who at times is assigned to complete an evaluation of a child or adolescent. After all, children and adolescents are not little adults!

While some of them may sound mature, their brains are not fully developed, which means they are deficient in critical thinking skills and emotional regulation and they still have a strong tendency to be impulsive and risk-taking. In general, adolescents are at high risk for making decisions and choices that are not thought out given that they are hormonally imbalanced and strongly socially influenced by peers and social media.

Besides the cognitive development issues, assessing adolescents and children has other challenges. Smaller children and those patients with intellectual disability may be unable to comprehend abstract assessment questions. There is also a significant prevalence of unmedicated attention deficit hyperactivity disorder (ADHD) or "bounce-back" evidenced by inattention and/or hyperactivity requiring repetition of questions. If not for the inattention, there is a high likelihood that the child or adolescent is coerced to be there, which means resistance or refusal in participation and emotional reactivity to the statements of the caregiver or collateral source. The clinician often must take behavioral steps to simplify the questions and manage the emotional climate to complete the interview and factually substantiate whether criteria are met.

While the clinician will likely use the same interview form, the admission criteria for children and adolescents are generally the same for adults with one addition: behavior. Besides suicidal ideation, homicidal ideation, and psychosis, a child or adolescent can be admitted for out of control, risky behavior that appears to be a danger to themselves or others. Some of the out of control behavior may be evident as a valid immediate safety risk, but much of the appearance of safety risk is dependent on the context painted by a caregiver or a collateral source.

The validity of the context can be tainted by pathology. There can be family pathology such as chaotic enmeshment with poor emotional boundaries and inconsistent parenting that erupts into a therapy session, disrupting the structure of the interview and possibly causing a disruption in the admitting or emergency departments. Furthermore, while the collateral of the caregiver can be quite valid and factual, there are other times when the problem is more the caregiver's pathological reaction than any actual behavior by the child or adolescent patient. If the caregiver evidences personality disorder traits, the interview can evolve into being more about the emotional issues of the caregiver rather than the reasons the patient is there for assessment. The clinician is therefore challenged in pathological situations to be emotionally detached and focused on substantiating clinical facts and whether criteria are met.

One other matter that can complicate or challenge the clinician in interviewing children and adolescents is that of legal compliance. Logically, the first compliance matter is that the guardian gives permission for the assessment and possible admission. However, the predominant legal matter is mandatary reporting of homicidal ideation, abuse, and neglect. One less frequently occurring matter is the privacy right of older adolescents such as under US regulation 42 CFR when an adolescent reports drug use. One more rare complication is when a sixteen- or seventeen-year-old presents alone requesting an assessment for substance use; they do not require guardian consent to be interviewed and admitted.

This chapter explores the variations in assessing children and adolescents. It reviews adjustments that clinicians may need to make to deal with those variations. It highlights the general legal parameters and obligations. A section of vignettes illustrates application of the concepts.

INTERVIEWING CONSIDERATIONS

As discussed in chapter 3, the child or adolescent is likely to be coerced to be in the interview, which will engender an emotional encounter. Adding to the emotion of merely being there, the patient will likely have had a tumultuous few hours or days prior to coming into the interview. Some of the tumult may have included conflict and argument with the caretaker. The patient will likely demonstrate defensiveness because of the vulnerability and intrusiveness.

The clinician can de-escalate the situation by utilizing the transactional analysis approach as discussed in chapter 3 and by using the modified boredom approach discussed in chapter 6; the clinician demonstrates the appearance of respect on an emotional level.[1] The child/adolescent patient is likely to reduce the level of defensiveness because the modified boredom tone tends to emit a lack of shock and is less likely to come across as patronization.

Besides the defensiveness, the child or adolescent may have a lower cognitive development level to comprehend and be able to give a valid answer to the more abstract questions. The clinician may have to revise some wording of questions to get valid answers.

The clinician will see a high prevalence of ADHD in interviews with children and adolescents. This is common when the presenting problem is disruptive behavior at school. The clinician may have to ask questions repeatedly and patiently because the patient's medication has metabolized out of the body or the patient has not been compliant with it; the patient is not necessarily being oppositional but is inattentive due to the disorder. Most of these ADHD cases will not meet criteria for inpatient admission and can be referred to outpatient levels of care.

THE IMMEDIATE SAFETY RISK

It bears mentioning that the overall standard for admission to inpatient is the same as adults: "an immediate safety risk" where the patient is a danger to themselves or others. For the adolescent and child, what constitutes an immediate safety risk is expanded in some categories.

Suicidal Ideation

Suicidal ideation is the first area of immediate safety risk. An adolescent with an attempt or specific plan in the past forty-eight hours continues to meet InterQual criteria as an immediate safety risk for inpatient admission. However, a child younger than age twelve with suicidal ideation and no plan is frequently considered to be an immediate safety risk and meeting inpatient criteria.[2]

Homicidal Ideation

Homicidal ideation is the next area of immediate safety risk. As with adults, homicidal ideation with a plan in the previous forty-eight hours is typically the standard for immediate safety risk and admission to inpatient. However, this area is expanded with physical aggression and property destruction.

The context of the patient's aggression will usually either be the school setting or the home setting. The report of the aggression will likely be given by one or more collateral sources that include (1) school officials, (2) referring mental health professionals, and (3) the parental figure present with the patient. The aggressive adolescent or child in such cases is frequently going to evidence denial about the behavior that can be manifested as refusal to cooperate with the interview or significant minimization of their behaviors earlier within the allowable time frame.

An exception to the matter of denial is in the case of a lower-intellectual-functioning patient. When it comes to younger children or adolescents with intellectual disability/mental retardation, there is the likelihood that the patient is incapable of understanding the questions. The patient may give some basic correlating affirmations, but such reports of homicidal ideation are completely dependent upon the caregiver, especially if the patient is non-verbal. Regardless of intellectual functioning, the physical aggression/homicidal ideation is frequently interpreted within the framework of whether the caretaker expresses confidence or a lack of confidence of being able to keep the patient and others safe in the home.

Psychosis

Psychosis is less common in children and adolescents than in adults. Nevertheless, there will be child and adolescent patients who report experiencing different positive symptoms (hallucinations, delusions) and will evidence negative symptoms of psychotic thought disorder that include thought blocking and disorganization in speech and behavior.

OUT OF CONTROL, RECKLESS, RISKY BEHAVIOR

With children and adolescents, the added category is behavioral in nature. Terms used can include out of control, risky, daredevil, and reckless. Examples of this behavior can include

1. a high degree of promiscuity that includes unprotected sex or sex with multiple partners;
2. fire-setting;
3. absentia, elopement, or running away for extended periods of time;
4. sexual abuse of younger children;
5. killing small animals or pets;
6. drug use;
7. impulsive engagement in "daredevil" or life-threatening behaviors; and
8. aggressive self-harm that can include head-banging or hitting self.

These behaviors in and of themselves do not necessarily merit inpatient admission. The essential task of the clinician is to establish that the patient's behavior immediately jeopardizes the safety of the patient or others. Part of the process of establishing the risk includes documentation of specific behaviors, their frequency, and when they last happened. Furthermore, the intellectual level of the patient should be considered especially when it comes to self-harming behavior, as admission to a specialized unit with behavior analysis is frequently indicated.[3] Establishment of the immediate safety risk for admission for behavioral reasons in these cases may need to involve extended consultation with a psychiatrist prior to making treatment recommendations.

Like homicidal ideation, context is significant regarding the parental figure's ability to keep the patient and other members of the household safe. The functional abilities and the resources of the parental figures and the vulnerabilities of the other household members must be considered.[4] On the other hand, the parental figure may fail to establish that dangerous behavior happened within the designated period for determining an immediate safety risk (usually three days): dangerous behavior that happened seven days prior to the assessment does not meet inpatient admission criteria.

ASSETS AND LIABILITIES OF THE CAREGIVER IN THE ASSESSMENT PROCESS

The typical interview with a child or adolescent will be conducted with a parental figure or caretaker. The parental figure or caretaker could include biological parents, adoptive parents, grandparents, guardians, foster parents, group home staff, and social workers.

The parental figure/caregiver is an integral part of the assessment to provide collateral information. They frequently have much to offer in describing behaviors, quotation statements, and the frequency/duration of concerning behaviors. As illustrated in vignette #3 in chapter 4, caregivers sometimes bring substantiating evidence in the forms of cellphone video/pictures and online posts, as well as written notes or drawings. In the case of lower-intellectual-functioning and non-verbal patients (who are in quadrants I or IV in the curve of ability as discussed in chapters 3 and 6), they are the sole source of information.

However, caregivers can also impede and interfere in the interview. One impediment is when the caregiver shares their own personal problems that may be irrelevant to the patient's behaviors. Second, the caretaker can be circumstantial in thought and make the interview all about them versus the patient. Third, the caretaker and patient may play out their relationship dynamics in the form of an argument and the assessment is turned into a family session with the clinician potentially triangulated in between them, which lengthens and potentially disrupts the interview. Furthermore, the caretaker may indeed have psychopathology that is driving family drama and that makes the patient look like the problem when it is not essentially the case. However, a silver lining to seeing the caregiver's interference is identification of possible precipitants to the patient's presenting problems.

The assessment of adolescents in the presence of their parents can be complex when there is chaotic enmeshment and poor boundaries. As illustrated in vignette #8 in chapter 3, a patient can become immediately reactive to the disclosures of the caretaker and an argument can ensue, disrupting the intent of the interview and creating a disturbance in the department. The clinician is thrust into the role of a family therapist to re-establish order. When the assessment appears to be evolving into a family session between the caretaker and the patient, the clinician can do the following to get the interview back on track:

1. Redirect either the patient or caregiver(s) to the waiting area.
2. Meet the child/adolescent alone to review questions of abuse, drug/alcohol activity, sexual involvement, sexual/gender identity, suicidal and homicidal thoughts, etc., seeking any inconsistencies from earlier in the interview.
3. Meet privately with the caregiver(s) to allow them to report their concerns.

At times, both the patient and the caretakers are embarrassed and hesitant to talk about matters, especially when adolescents tend to value privacy. They also can be reactive to each other as part of their conflict. Separation allows the clinician to be able to get the facts and then determine whether criteria are met (this is demonstrated in vignette #9 of this chapter).

In the cases of caregiver pathology, the "Munchausen syndrome by proxy" construct can be applicable. The caregiver's personality disorder traits include an inability to cope with the stress of parenting, and they interpret the child or adolescent's behavior in an "all or nothing" manner as the problem, when the opposite is true. The caregiver may also be the instigator of the antecedent problems in the household and is projecting them upon the patient. The child's behavior also may be natural reactions to the parent's instigation. One example of such a situation is when such a caretaker verbally abuses the child or adolescent patient and the patient reacts; the child is argumentative and therefore "misbehaving" in the eyes of the caretaker. Another example is that of an adolescent being physically defensive toward the caretaker's physical abuse (or inappropriate corporal punishment) that the caretaker therefore reports as the patient being "assaultive."[5] When interviewed separately from the caretaker, the patient may give a report that suggests such a situation. The assessment clinician is not necessarily going to have an immediate intervention at that moment, but they should make a child protective services (CPS) report. If the patient and caretaker (with apparent psychopathology) have a physical fight in the admitting department, it might be appropriate to take one or more of the following steps:

1. Admit the patient for safety if other clinical criteria are met in the assessment.
2. Call law enforcement to intervene.
3. Call CPS and immediately report the incident.
4. Arrange for an emergency shelter placement if inpatient admission criteria are not met.

LEGAL OBLIGATIONS

Even if the assessment does not evolve into a family session, given the legal obligations, it is crucial that the clinician attempt to meet with the patient alone to get impartial information and respect the patient's privacy. With privacy, a child or adolescent tends to be more open about abuse, neglect, and human trafficking. Privacy also allows for greater compliance with federal law 42 CFR when it comes to drug use.

Abuse

As discussed earlier, abuse and trauma questions are typical components of structured assessment interviews. The abuse categories are emotional/verbal, physical, sexual, and neglect. Human trafficking has become of increasing concern in the twenty-first century. Insurance reviewers may ask about abuse and trauma histories as part of the prior authorizations.

Developmental limitations are a concern in assessing trauma. It may not seem obvious, but the wording a clinician uses to inquire about such possible abuse may need to be tailored for the patient's developmental level. Older adolescents and middle-school-aged children can be asked in an abstract manner such as: *Have you ever been physically, verbally, or sexually abused or neglected?* With younger children, the clinician may have to use more concrete wording, such as:

- Has a grown up ever hit you and really hurt you?
- Has someone ever done "bad touch" to you?
- Has anyone touched you inappropriately in your private places?
- Have you ever gone hungry for days or not had enough clothing?

The tone of voice in asking abuse questions to a child should be gentle, kind, respectful, and business-like. It is a safe assumption that the interview has been scary and uncomfortable for the child, especially if the caretaker was critical and judgmental of the patient in front of them and to their face. With respect to the trauma-informed care paradigm, asking a child the abuse questions in such situations can be equally alienating and traumatizing, especially if there has been some abuse. With younger patients, clinician tone of voice can make the difference in garnering cooperation versus the child shutting down and being silent.

The clinician can engage in some correlation of factuality with the caretaker before or after asking the patient. Example of questions to the caretaker on abuse and neglect are as follows:

- Has the household ever been the subject of a CPS investigation?
- When?
- What were the circumstances?
- Is CPS currently involved in any capacity?
- Do you have the phone number to the current CPS worker?

Visual observation is part of abuse assessment. A child or adolescent's withdrawal (e.g., poor eye contact, lack of participation) may be an indicator of fear or emotional abuse. Physical abuse may be present when there are noticeable scars, bruises, burns, or cuts. Neglect may be indicated when a child presents as being underweight and having poor hygiene. If a youth has a sexually transmitted infection, this also could indicate sexual abuse. Furthermore, signs of regressive behaviors suggesting possible sexual abuse include thumb-sucking, bed-wetting, painful urination, encopresis (defecation in clothes or places other than the toilet), and/or difficulty walking or sitting. The clinician should document any disclosures and observations.

It is another safe assumption that the assessment clinician is considered a mandated reporter in all jurisdictions. Therefore, any abuse of a child confirmed or disconfirmed by a caregiver must be reported to CPS in the state where the patient resides. If a clinician is unsure whether a disclosure necessitates reporting, they should consult with a supervisor.

If a supervisor is unavailable, it is a safe practice simply to make the report. It is a typical policy of state protective service agencies that they should be the ones in vague situations to determine if further investigation is warranted and that the clinician should not make an independent decision. Good faith reporting does not make for legal penalty; however, failure to report can lead to licensure board or other legally applicable sanction.

Trafficking

Human trafficking of adults and youth has become a growing concern in multiple domains including legal, psychological, and physical safety. It is becoming an increasingly held clinical standard to screen for trafficking. Possible signs that youth may be involved in human trafficking include

- avoidance of direct eye contact;
- nervousness, shyness, or fear of speaking;
- a caregiver who refuses to allow clinician to speak with the youth alone;
- physical injuries;
- tattoos on teenagers;
- scripted, memorized, or mechanical recitation of medical history; and
- indicators of sexual abuse (see previous section on abuse).[6]

42 CFR, Part 2

To encourage minors to be more forthcoming with their substance abuse, a federal law was written to protect the confidentiality of patients seeking substance use treatment. It applies to programs that provide substance abuse treatment that are federally assisted. Such facilities cannot release any patient information regarding substance use treatment without written consent, including all ages.[7] In the context of assessment, this means a clinician cannot share with caregivers the youth's reporting of substance abuse unless the clinician has the child/adolescent's written consent on a "release of information" form; the clinician can share mental health information, but not substance use information. The only exception to this rule would be a mandatory reporting situation in the context of a medical/psychiatric emergency that poses an immediate threat to the patient's health.

Consent

Consent is a legal matter with children and adolescent patients. There are two stages of consent: first to do the assessment and then to do the admission. Normally when biological parents or guardians bring the patient in, they will sign permission for assessment upon entry to the admitting department. If admission is recommended, then the parent or guardian will need to sign a permission to treat or admit.

Both stages are relevant, especially when the patient is a ward of the state. It will be necessary to get permission from the state social worker or designated state representative for both assessment and admission.

A youth under the age of sixteen years must be accompanied by their guardian to be assessed or consent must be obtained with a phone call prior to evaluation. The exception to this rule is if the minor seeking an assessment is doing so for the purpose of receiving treatment for substance use; in this case, the guardian does not need to be present nor does the clinician need to obtain consent via phone. Although a sixteen- or seventeen-year-old, as well as the aforementioned youth seeking an assessment for substance abuse, can consent for themselves to be evaluated (should the clinician decide the individual needs to be admitted), a youth under the age of sixteen must have consent from their guardian prior to admission whether it be for substance use or mental health. When the guardian declines to consent, the clinician and physician must decide whether involuntary admission is indicated.

Adolescents sixteen years and older can consent for evaluation and for admission. It follows that they also can refuse to consent to admission even if the caretaker gives consent. If the adolescent refuses to consent, it is then incumbent upon the psychiatrist to determine whether the patient should be placed on a seventy-two-hour hold.[8]

VIGNETTES

The following eight case vignettes are based on the clinical experience of the authors with children, adolescents, and their caretakers. Only vignette #8 has dialogue; the remainder are limited to the discussion of case details with the treatment recommendations.

Vignette #1: Fourteen-Year-Old Female

A fourteen-year-old was brought by her mother to a psychiatric hospital admitting department. The patient reported feeling depressed and that she had been having suicidal thoughts. She and her boyfriend had broken up ten days prior to the assessment, and she has become estranged from her friends in the process. She has been isolating in her room, and her grades have been declining. The youth reports sleep and appetite impairment. She reported having had a previous suicide gesture approximately six months prior in which she held a knife to her wrists but was interrupted by her friend. She denied having a suicide plan, but she did not feel that she would be safe. The treatment recommendation was that the patient be admitted inpatient.

Vignette #2: Seventeen-Year-Old Male

The patient had presented to the admitting department reporting substance abuse and anger issues. He had been fired that day from his job, had an argument about it with his parents, and then was kicked out of the house. The patient was tearful and said he was really upset by his father calling him a "Worthless idiot." The patient added that his father was always putting him down and had even told him to "Go kill yourself!" The patient revealed a plan to "beat his father into submission" tonight after his parents went to bed with a hammer that he had access to.

The treatment recommendation was that the patient be admitted inpatient. Furthermore, the clinician needed to call CPS due to the disclosure of emotional abuse and neglect and then make the duty to warn notifications to the father (intended victim) and to the relevant law enforcement agencies.

Vignette #3: Fifteen-Year-Old Male

A mother brought the patient to a psychiatric hospital admitting department reporting, "The boy is pushing my last button." When the clinician asked a clarifying question, the mother bellowed, "Let me start with his school work; he doesn't listen to his teachers and refuses to finish assignments at school or when he gets home." The teen told the clinician he has been acting up in school because it is hard to concentrate in a noisy classroom and he does not remember the assignments when he gets home. The mother also reported that the patient gets into verbal and mild physical altercations (pushing/shoving) with his twin brother that mostly occur when she is busy with her "work from home" job; she is facing possible employee discipline due to the numerous disruptions. The patient said that his ADHD medication was not working, and his mother went on in detail that she herself has recently been put on a new psychotropic medication and discussed the side effects and benefits in detail.

The clinician allowed the patient's mother to vent and redirected the mother and patient back to the questions. The patient had denied suicidal ideation, homicidal ideation, and psychosis. This appeared to be a matter of the patient having symptoms of ADHD impacting both in the home and school. The treatment recommendation was to refer the patient to outpatient services.

Vignette #4: Seven-Year-Old Male

A concerned mother brought her seven-year-old son reporting that he was engaging in dangerous behaviors. She said that he "doesn't think before he does things," is reckless, and has "no fear." She reported that he has been climbing out his second-story bedroom window in the middle of the night. Furthermore, he wandered the previous evening to their neighbor's houses, knocking on doors and trying to get in.

The mother also reported that the patient has anger issues. He could be violent in terms of breaking things at home and exhibiting aggression toward the family dog and his younger three-year-old sister. Last night, he pushed his sister off the couch causing bruises, and he kicked the dog. The patient has been in outpatient services, and the mother reported his current therapist diagnosed him with "impulse control disorder." The treatment recommendation was for the patient to be admitted inpatient.

Vignette #5: Sixteen-Year-Old Female

A sixteen-year-old girl's parents brought her in for assessment reporting that she had been putting herself in precarious circumstances. The teenager had been staying at her aunt's house the last two days since a series of incidents. At least two weeks ago, she had started chatting with older men online and had been sending them nude pictures. She had also been experimenting with illegal drugs and binge drinking alcohol on the weekends. She ran away for five days after her father reprimanded her. She was found by her parents passed out in a car with an older man in a mall parking lot. The clinician spoke with the teenager alone after talking to her and her parents as a group and then the parents alone. The parents inquired what their daughter had reported to the clinician alone in terms of her drug and alcohol use; the teen had not signed a release of information.

The clinician had to say to the parents that unless their daughter signed a release of information, the clinician was unable to answer questions about substance use under federal law 42 CFR, Part 2. Nevertheless, the clinician staffed the case with the next psychiatrist on rotation, and the treatment recommendation was inpatient admission. The patient agreed to voluntary admission.

Vignette #6: Fifteen-Year-Old Female from a Residential Facility

A fifteen-year-old female was referred to a psychiatric hospital by a residential facility due to "out of control" aggression and self-injurious behavior. She was reported to use contraband to cut her arms and throat to the extent of requiring bandaging but not stiches. The patient also had been engaging in fistfights with peers. Finally, the teen was observed attempting to "stab a staff member" with a plastic cutlery knife at lunch on the day of the referral; she was stopped by a peer before she could assault the employee. The treatment recommendation was that the patient be admitted inpatient.

Vignette #7: Seventeen-Year-Old Female Presenting without Parent or Caretaker

A seventeen-year-old female came alone to a psychiatric hospital for assessment reporting using multiple substances, engaging in petty theft, and self-injurious behavior. There was no need for consent from a parent or guardian given her age. The patient reported she had been occasionally smoking marijuana, drinking beer, and had used Xanax a couple times. She said she shoplifted a sandwich and a soft drink from a gas station because she did not have any money. The patient reported that she will sometimes cut on her upper thigh with a razor to deal with her anxiety when not drinking, using marijuana, or taking the Xanax.

The treatment recommendation was outpatient services due to the lack of suicidal ideation, homicidal ideation, psychosis, and daredevil behavior (the shoplifting was risky but necessarily not life-threatening). At hearing the recommendation, the patient said that she was not interested in getting treatment and left.

Vignette #8: The Transgender Youth with Opposing Parent

The registration papers said that the patient was a fourteen-year-old female. It was scribbled at the top of the first page that the patient wanted to be "Vick" but "her proper name was Victoria" and her mother did not want her being called "Vick." The reason for assessment on the form was "Out of control behavior and she said that she had wanted to kill herself." A chart review prior to the interview indicated that the patient had no previous admissions at this facility.

The clinician called into the waiting room for "Victoria." A middle-aged female and what appeared to be a biological female adolescent with short hair dressed in masculine clothing got up and came to the door. The clinician led them to an interview room and beckoned them inside. As the clinician was walking to his computer desk and sitting down, he introduced himself.

Clinician: Hello, my name is Dave. I am a social worker and I have been with the hospital twenty years. I will do your assessment tonight. The interview is confidential but under state laws, if someone reports that they want to kill or hurt someone, I must do what is called a duty to warn, and if someone reports abuse or neglect, I may have to make a report because I am a mandated reporter. Otherwise, what is said here will stay here. It says that your name is Victoria, what would you like to be called?

Patient: Vick.

Mom: I don't like her using that name.

Clinician: Okay . . . I understand. Well, hospital policy is that we call patients what they prefer to be called. So, Vick, why did your mother bring you here to be interviewed?

Patient: I don't know . . . probably because I said that I wanted to kill myself today?

Clinician: You are Ms. M? Correct?

Mom: Yes.

Clinician: Why did you need to bring your daughter to be assessed tonight?

Mom: She said today that she was going to kill herself.

Clinician: Did she tell you how she was going to do it?

Mom: She said that she was going to grab some pills.

The clinician had software that allowed for flexibility in interview sequence. While not in normal order, the clinician ran through the following sections with the patient and the mother in the room together:

- *suicidal ideation,*
- *homicidal ideation/aggression,*
- *legal history,*
- *depressive symptoms,*
- *treatment history,*
- *community providers,*
- *medical history, and*
- *developmental history.*

Clinician: This is where the interview works better when I interview kids and their parents separately. I get impartial or at least better answers to questions. So, Ms. M, what I would like to do is have you go out into the waiting room, and we will change places in about fifteen minutes. Will that be okay?

Mom: Okay.

The clinician resumed the interview after verifying that the patient's mother was in the waiting room.

Clinician: Okay, Vick, I plan to take about fifteen minutes unless you have more to talk about. I am going to start with the abuse and neglect questions. Do you consider yourself to have been the victim of verbal or emotional abuse?

Patient: No.

Clinician: Do you consider yourself to be the victim of physical abuse?

Patient: No.

Clinician: Have you been sexually abused? Touched inappropriately?

Patient: Yes. A cousin touched me when I was seven.

Clinician: Did you report it?

Patient: Yes.

Clinician: Did CPS get involved?

Patient: Yes.

Clinician: Have you been the victim of neglect? For example, you have gone without food and clothes and heat?

Patient: No.

Clinician: Have you experienced any other trauma that gives you nightmares or continues to bother you?

Patient: No.

Clinician: Okay, this is the sexual history section. I always tell people this is none of my personal business, but they want to know this information. How do you identify your gender?

Patient: I'm a dude.

Clinician: Do you have preferred pronouns?

Patient: He/him.

Clinician: How do you define your sexual orientation?

Patient: I'm straight.

Clinician: Do you consider yourself to be sexually active? Are you having sex with people?

Patient: No.

Clinician: Do you consider yourself to be practicing safe sex?

Patient: I don't know.

Clinician: We usually call no sex as being safe sex. Can we put yes in this box?

Patient: Sure.

Clinician: Moving on. This is the domestic violence section. Are you currently in a relationship?

Patient: Yes.

Clinician: Do you feel safe in your relationship?

Patient: Yes.

Clinician: In the past year, have you been hit, kicked, or physically hurt by someone?

Patient: No.

The clinician then went through the substance use and mental status sections.

The patient

- *denied any substance use;*
- *was oriented to reality in all four spheres (time, person, place, and activity);*
- *denied feeling paranoid, hearing voices, or experiencing visual hallucinations;*
- *described their mood as "irritated"; and*
- *evidenced logical thought content.*

After completion of the interview questions, the clinician asked the patient an open-ended question.

Clinician: Vick, is there anything you want to talk about without your mother in the room?

Patient: Am I going to be admitted?

Clinician: I can't answer that yet. I need to finish talking to your mother and then talk to a doctor. Any other questions?

Patient: No.

Clinician: Okay, Vick. I'll have you go into the waiting room and I'll talk with your mother.

The clinician had the patient go out into the waiting room and called the mother back.

Clinician: Ms. M. I asked your child about trauma, substance use, sexual history, and did the mental status exam. Has CPS ever been in your home to investigate anything?

Mother: Yes, she said that a cousin touched her, and it was investigated.

Clinician: Have you ever had to redirect your child for anything of a sexual nature?

Mother: Like what?

Clinician: Like, have they ever posted inappropriate pictures of themselves online?

Mother: No.

Clinician: Have you caught them with any tobacco, alcohol, or drugs that were not prescribed?

Mother: No.

Clinician: Is there anything that you are specifically looking for tonight?

Mother: I am worried about her safety, and I am afraid that she is going to hurt herself. I want her hospitalized.

Clinician: Is there anything else you would like to talk about?

Mother: It really hurts me that she is calling herself a boy and that she is calling herself Vick.

Clinician: I do not have any easy answers for that. All I can say is that it can be tough for some people when a family member, especially a child, comes out as transgender. I'll go ahead and call a doctor and be back with you shortly.

The clinician staffed the case with the next psychiatrist on rotation, who accepted the patient for admission since there was substantiation that the patient had reported being suicidal with a plan. The clinician then called the house manager to get permission to move other patients around to accommodate the patient in a private room.

When the clinician gave report to the nurse, the clinician made it clear that the patient's chosen name was Vick and had preferred pronouns "he" and "him." The clinician also discussed Vick's mother as being opposed to the patient's identifying as transgender.

The clinician had to balance between the patient's right to be called by the patient's chosen name and the mother's opposition to the patient's transgender identity. Interviewing the patient and mother separately, especially when covering the gender questions, was efficient and avoided potential arguments that could have erupted if the mother had remained in the room the whole time. The clinician talked to Vick in the same manner as any other patient but also empathized with Vick's mother. However, once Vick identified as male, the clinician started using gender-neutral terms like "child" and "they/them." The clinician empathized with the mother's feelings in a neutral manner without judgment. The clinician showed respect for both Vick and his mom while avoiding getting triangulated in the conflict.

CONCLUDING THOUGHTS

While the interview questions are going to be the same, the assessment of a child or adolescent is, in a word, different from that of an adult and can be challenging even for the seasoned clinician. It can be a balancing act to manage the various elements discussed in this chapter. It can demand vigilant focus to assemble a factual picture of the situation, determine whether the appropriate criteria are validly met, and meet all legal obligations regarding abuse, neglect, and privacy. The clinician may have to attend to the patient's cognitive level and ability to comprehend the answers and clarify whether their answers are valid responses. There are assessments of children or adolescents that can have a lot of moving parts of conflict and distortion created by caregivers.

With the standard set of abuse and neglect questions in the standard structured interview, there is certainty that the clinician will be mandated to file CPS reports, especially in the pathological situations. Patients will make statements that are both clear and vague indications of abuse necessitating CPS notification. To borrow a meme from a television show, "The truth is out there"—outside the assessment room—and the clinician will not be able to investigate it. Given the potential legal consequences of not reporting in most jurisdictions, it is safer for the clinician to make the report in good faith to CPS who has the legislated prerogative to make any such determinations.

In the more chaotic and dysfunctional situations, the clinician must demonstrate assertiveness and directiveness with both the patient and caregiver to maintain order. Either the caregiver or patient can instigate drama that lengthens the time required to finish the interview. The clinician can use a "script" or prepared statement in a modified bored tone: "I think I need to interview you separately." The clinician should move to separate the arguing caretaker and child or adolescent sooner than later in the interview.

There is a chance that some of the more pathological caretakers are also savvy of treatment terminology and processes and are intimidating toward new clinicians. Savvy, pathological caretakers tend to use hospitals as ways to punish the patient and may fabricate indisputable information that criteria have been met. The clinician who sets limits with them may be subject to demands to talk with supervisors, personal attacks in front of audiences, and various threats to make complaints to file grievances or call government authorities. Such demands and threats are instigations of drama by the caretaker (may feel like abuse) and are emotionally draining if not genuinely terrifying for the new clinician. This is one of those baptisms by fire that new clinicians are thrown into and that lead to burnout if the clinician cannot adjust. The transactional analysis and assertiveness strategies discussed in chapter 4 and to be discussed in chapter 12 can cue the clinician how to *respond* (and not react) to the patient or pathological caregiver as they both may be highly emotionally and acting in child state or an immature manner.

NOTES

1. The clinician should avoid tangents by avoiding making statements about how much the clinician respects the client/patient. Respect should be embedded in the

emotional transaction. Given the technical focus of this book, there has been limited discussion of gender identity issues, but respecting the identity of an adolescent who disclosed other than cisgender identity using the chosen name versus the legal name can be one key to de-escalation and getting the interview on track with valid answers.

2. This is according to the 2013 InterQual criteria available to the writers, which was published by the McKesson Corporation. It serves to repeat that InterQual continues to be a proprietary intellectual property and requires subscription to use the latest edition. Managed care organizations, in the experience of the authors, have used criteria close to this.

3. A child or adolescent patient can engage in severe head-banging and self-harming that requires observation and analysis by trained behavioral analysts as to cause.

4. A parent may be in a wheelchair and physically unable to manage the aggression of a child. The parent may be the only caretaker in the house and cannot supervise the patient satisfactorily to maintain safety. If some of the daredevil/reckless behavior puts the whole household in danger (e.g., fire-setting), then inpatient may be indicated.

5. Parents will often press charges against the patients in such situations.

6. If human trafficking is suspected, the assessment clinician should talk with the youth privately to ask more specific questions such as if they are required to work or face physical punishment, if they are forced to have sex, if they work without pay, if they are threatened with violence for trying to leave, and/or if they are kept from contacting friends or family. Furthermore, the assessment clinician can inquire if their residency or legal status is being threatened. Should trafficking be confirmed or suspected, the assessment clinician should reach out to their superior to see about potentially contacting a legal authority. This encounter would be more likely to happen as a field interview in a hospital emergency room as a part of treatment for a medical condition as opposed to a psychiatric hospital admission department. The clinician will need to have the support of the emergency department physician and security personnel to interview the patient alone if the caretaker starts to escalate. The physician may also need to place the patient on a seventy-two-hour hold to allow security and police to intervene should the escalated caretaker try to elope with the patient from the emergency department before the clinician can privately interview the patient.

7. When substance use is part of the reason for presentation, caregivers tend to have a prior knowledge and appreciation of the patient's use but not necessarily the extent. It is the experience of the authors that adolescents are more forthright about their substance use in front of caretakers especially if that is the reason for assessment.

8. Typically, the patient can only be placed on a hold if the patient is suicidal or homicidal. The adolescent patient whose reason for presentation is merely running away and refusing to sign in voluntarily will be referred to a partial or outpatient program. This can be a difficult, emotional experience for the clinician when a caretaker outwardly laments about how concerned they are for their child. Savvy caretakers have added information that the patient has made a suicidal statement (that the patient will deny) to up the ante and create substantial grounds for a seventy-two-hour hold.

Chapter 8

Substance Use Assessment

Since the mid-twentieth century, substance use has been identified as a public health problem and the medical profession has been consigned to treat it. Furthermore, there has been considerable attention given to the matter of "dual diagnosis" when there is co-morbid psychiatric and substance use symptoms. Substance use treatment has evolved to be delivered along a continuum of care due to the level of severity or intensity of symptoms. From most intense to least intense it is as follows:

- Inpatient detox
- Residential
- Partial hospitalization
- Intensive outpatient
- Outpatient

Inpatient detox focuses on assisting the patient who has been heavily using alcohol, opioids, or benzodiazepines to get safely through withdrawal through a protocol of medication. Residential treats patients who are not having severe detox symptoms and who need a treatment milieu to change mindsets and behavior patterns. The partial hospitalization and intensive outpatient levels treat patients who do not meet criteria for admission to inpatient detox or residential but who have symptomology or use patterns that are disruptive to daily functioning or that are otherwise unmanageable.[1] The outpatient level of care is indicated when a patient's use pattern is not disruptive to daily functioning.

What complicates the discussion of the treatment continuum is substance-induced psychosis. Amphetamine and synthetic drugs cause heavy users to present in severe, active psychosis. They do not detox like those who had been using opiates, benzodiazepines, or alcohol, but they can present as severely psychotic as depicted in quadrant IV of the curve of ability (discussed in chapters 3 and 5) that may require inpatient treatment for the safety of the patient and others.

The typical psychiatric hospital offers a continuum of substance use treatment that includes inpatient detox, partial hospitalization, and intensive outpatient.[2] Depending on the severity of the use history and motivation, patients completing detox may be referred to residential for intense treatment for a period of twenty-eight days or longer. The American Society of Addiction Medicine (ASAM) scale (discussed subsequently) is used to determine whether criteria have been met for residential treatment. Those discharging patients who are not meeting ASAM criteria for residential can then be offered partial hospitalization or intensive outpatient.

Substance use treatment is a discipline or specialty that typically requires attainment of unique training and licensure or certification. There are many individuals with addiction or dual diagnosis whose symptomology reaches a crisis point and out of personal motivation seek treatment or have been mandated to get assessment and screening.[3] Regardless of the motivation, the assessment clinician, who does not necessarily have the special training or licensure, is still in the position to be the doorkeeper for admission to such treatment by specialists.

The assessment clinician will eventually be practiced in asking substance use screening questions, because they are part of the standard interview script. However, when the presenting problem is substance abuse, there are challenges to getting a thorough, valid assessment and referring a patient to the appropriate level of care when the presenting problem is indeed substance use. Seeking substance use treatment is often difficult for the addicted patient in the first place and, as a result, they inaccurately report their use. Furthermore, addicted patients present with different levels of psychiatric symptomology and cognitive impairment which contributes to inaccurate reporting. Third, an inexperienced clinician can be unaware of the plethora of drug types as well as their effects and withdrawal potentials. Furthermore, assessment clinicians must screen for potential medical crises related to substance use and withdrawal.

This chapter seeks to orient the reader in substance use assessment as to the level of care determination. It will cover taking the substance use history and the two primary detox assessment instruments. It will then review the scope of substance types, the criteria for admission, and making treatment recommendations.

TAKING THE HISTORY

There is an inherent tension between the clinician's pursuit of getting an accurate substance use history and the patient's reluctance and probable cognitive impairment due to symptomology or intoxication. Patient reluctance can come from negative emotion or an agenda to be admitted.[4] Such negative emotions include shame, embarrassment, ambivalence, irritability, and fear of the withdrawal symptoms themselves. Many patients are embarrassed about their reasons for use and their triggers for relapse. On the other hand, the agenda to be admitted usually produces exaggerated reports of use and detox symptoms.[5] The intoxicated patient may also present as a poor historian with cognitive impairment and emotional instability.

Considering these, the clinician should foster a safe space of non-judgment for the individual to describe how long they have been using (i.e., duration), how often they are using (i.e., frequency), how much they are using per use (i.e., amount), and last use; how these appear in a typical interview is depicted in table 8.1.[6]

Potential Medical Crises Due to Intoxication and Detox

Equally important is assessing the degree of intoxication, withdrawal severity, and history of complicated withdrawal (seizures or delirium tremens). In intoxication or detox cases, screening for physical symptoms takes priority over mental status.[7] Some independent psychiatric hospitals will send patients with a blood alcohol level of 0.300 or higher out for medical clearance. Intoxicated patients presenting as drowsy, delirious, or unable to blow a breathalyzer result also should be sent for medical clearance to rule out overdose or alcohol poisoning.

The clinician should monitor the patient's condition throughout the interview. This includes awareness of medical history, vital signs, observed withdrawal symptoms, and physical complaints. In cases of high vital signs, the clinician should review symptoms with the designated nursing staff prior to assessment.

Use and Relapse Triggers

When taking the substance use history, the clinician should attempt to ascertain reasons for the substance use if the patient can articulate a response. There can be many precipitants to an individual's substance abuse or relapse. Ascertaining these precipitants will inform program staff as to the approach of relapse prevention. The following are common relapse triggers:

- Medical condition/pain condition
- History of prescribed pain medication
- Environmental stressors
    - Homelessness
    - Relational loss

Table 8.1. Typical Substance Use Question Grid

Substance	*Age First Used*	*Average Amount*	*Frequency*	*Routes Used*	*Last Used*	*Amount in Last Twenty-Four Hours*
Tobacco						
Alcohol						
Cannabis						
Cocaine						
Psychedelics						
Opiates						
Amphetamines						
Inhalants						
Synthetics						
Benzodiazepines						

  - Job loss
  - Traumatic event
- Self-medication
  - Depression
  - Anxiety
  - Trauma
  - Psychosis
- Social circle influence
- Genetic predisposition

SCOPE OF DRUG AND ALCOHOL TYPES

There are several types of drug and alcohol use, and the assessment clinician should have an appreciation of examples that fall into each type, effects on the body and mind, and the potential for withdrawal. This section reviews the categories in the following order: stimulants, psychedelics, opiates, and alcohol/benzodiazepines. It will discuss admission criteria in the case of each of these drug categories.

Stimulants

Stimulants are drugs that provide an energy boost and euphoric feelings. Stimulants include

- cocaine,
- methamphetamine (also known as Meth, Ice, Crank),
- over-the-counter diet pills,
- prescription attention deficit hyperactivity disorder medications (Adderall, Concerta, and Ritalin),[8] and
- MDMA/ecstasy.

Some stimulants are short acting like cocaine, while others are long lasting like methamphetamines. Stimulants tend to raise pulse and blood pressure and cause chest pain. If used in excess, there is a potential danger of cardiac arrest. The clinician should observe for elevated vital signs, diaphoresis (perspiration/sweating), rushed speech, and rapid movement and again refer the patient to qualified medical personnel if the patient presents as in medical distress. Abuse and dependence may cause insomnia several days in a row. Such extended insomnia can cause severe psychosis (hallucinations, paranoia, delusions, and disorganization). If there are any noticeable withdrawal symptoms from stimulants, they are mild and in the forms of tiredness, mood swings, body aches, sleep difficulty, and tremors/shakiness.

Synthetic and Psychedelic Drugs

Synthetic and psychedelic drugs tend to induce some level mood alteration and/or type of psychosis either by virtue of intoxication or insomnia. These substances include

- cannabis/marijuana,[9]
- psychedelics (PCP, LSD, mescaline, psilocybin mushrooms, DMT MDMA),
- inhalants (gasoline, epoxy, computer duster, ether),
- synthetic marijuana (Spice), and
- bath salts (synthetic stimulants).

Cannabis is the most used of these substances. It is technically classified as a hallucinogen; it alters mood, perception, and judgment. It is dependence-forming as regular use builds tolerance, requiring increased frequency to get the desired effect and prevent withdrawal. Its use transcends cultures, age groups, and socioeconomic groups. Its use has expanded beyond mere smoking as it is available to "vape" and in food items called "edibles." It is evolving in its social acceptance as it is becoming decriminalized and legally acceptable in an increasing number of jurisdictions for both medical and recreational use.

Psychedelics produce an altered mental status and psychosis. They have been historically used in natural forms by various people groups in spiritual practices. They developed secular popularity in the 1960s by the "hippie" generation. There is medical interest in using psychedelics in the treatment of anxiety, trauma, and depression. Psychedelics are available in both synthetic and natural forms.

The direct inhaling of aerosols and vapors from certain chemicals can produce euphoria but can cause acute psychosis and brain damage. Slang terms include "sniffing" or "huffing." In the North American context, such "inhalant" use has primarily been done by youth. It is not as common as the use of cannabis or psychedelics or synthetic drugs.

Opiates

Opiates are sedating in nature and can bring about a euphoric, pain-relieving experience for the user. Opiates include

- heroin,
- fentanyl,
- pain pills (i.e., Percocet, Darvocet, Oxycontin, hydrocodone, Vicodin), and
- opiate replacement drugs (i.e., Suboxone, methadone).

Opiates are dangerous due to the high potential of dependency and risk of overdose. Dependent users require higher amounts to avoid withdrawal and can easily overdose. A patient disclosing opiate use evidencing depressed vital signs and problems staying awake or focusing should be assessed by a qualified medical professional for medical clearance and possible stabilization.

Opiate withdrawal tends to be painful and severe with symptoms comparable to the flu. Withdrawal symptoms include

- vomiting,
- gastrointestinal upset,
- diarrhea,
- diaphoresis (perspiration),
- rhinorrhea (running nose),
- tremors,
- restlessness,
- joint pain,
- dilated eyes,
- frequent yawning,
- pulse rate greater than ninety beats per minute,
- goose bumps, and
- significant anxiety.

The severity of opiate withdrawal is determined through the Clinical Opiate Withdrawal Scale (COWS),[10] which will be discussed further.

The COWS worksheet is often integrated into software and hospital-constructed worksheets, but it is also readily available in the public domain on the internet. The answers are derived by taking the patient's vitals, objectively observing the relevant symptoms, and asking questions that can only be derived by self-report. The direct observable symptoms to input on the COWS worksheet are

- the number of times a patient yawns in the interview,
- goose bumps,
- dilated eyes,
- runny nose,
- tearing/watery eyes, and
- if a patient vomits in the interview or has evidenced vomiting.

COWS questions can include the following:

- Are you having any stomach cramps?
- Have you vomited or had diarrhea in the past few hours?
- Do you have any pain in your joints?

- How hard is it for you to sit still?
- Other than the fact that I am a total stranger asking intrusive questions, how anxious are you?[11]

Some patients seeking admission for opioid detox may not have any symptoms because they used just prior to arrival at the admitting or emergency department. To get admitted, they will often say that they are suicidal with a plan; otherwise, such patients not in detox and without suicidal ideation may have to wait and be reassessed after a few hours for the onset withdrawal symptoms.[12]

Alcohol and Benzodiazepines

Alcohol and benzodiazepines will be addressed together on account of their similar physical effects and withdrawal symptomology. Alcohol is a commonly available substance, while benzodiazepines are a controlled class of drug legally available only by prescription.

Alcohol

Alcohol comes in several potable categories that include beers or ales, wines, and distilled spirits (e.g., whiskey, vodka, gin, rum, tequila, brandy, liqueurs/cordials). Beers and ales are created by the direct fermentation of one or more grains. Wine is fermented fruit juice.[13] "Spirits" are created by distilling a form of fermented beer, wine, or sugar that evaporates water and concentrates alcohol content. The distilled spirits may be sold by themselves (whiskey, vodka, tequila, rum) or mixed with sweeteners and flavorings to make liqueurs.

Individuals with alcohol dependence issues, who are craving, and who or are desperate to use may consume non-potable forms of alcohol when potable forms are not available.[14] These non-potable forms include rubbing alcohol, hand sanitizer, mouthwash, cologne/aftershave, and aerosol disinfectant. These non-potable forms can be fatal in and of themselves but mostly have negative health effects.

Alcohol has sedating effects on the brain and body that includes slowed reaction times. Intoxication has a range of symptoms that include

- a loss of coordination, such as stumbling or swaying,
- flushing of the face,
- bloodshot eyes,
- louder speech than usual,
- slurred speech,

- clammy (or damp) skin,
- mood swings or personality changes, such as aggression or depression, and
- drowsiness.

Intoxicated individuals may show reduced self-control and judgment that include higher levels of impulsivity, poor boundaries, and socially inappropriate comments. The higher the intoxication,

- the more unsteady the balance,
- the slower the motor functions,[15]
- the more incoherent the speech,
- the higher the lack of inhibition, and
- the higher the impulsivity.

It follows that intoxicated individuals are at higher risk for suicidal and homicidal ideation or attempts. Furthermore, chronic, heavy consumption can have damaging physical effects.

As with opiates, an individual with chronic, heavy consumption patterns of alcohol develops tolerance. It requires increased amounts of alcohol to avoid going into detox and get the desired effect. Individuals with higher tolerance do not necessarily show the expected motor and speech impairments. It is distinctly possible that the person with high tolerance can continue to consume to the point of overdose (blood alcohol level = 0.400), which in this case is called "alcohol poisoning."

Alcohol withdrawal symptoms can include

- headache,
- body ache,
- gastrointestinal issues,
- vomiting,
- tremors/shakiness,
- disorientation,
- elevated vital signs,
- delirium tremens (a combination of psychosis and tremors), and
- seizures.

The withdrawal seizures are dangerous and potentially lethal. The clinician should screen for if a patient has a history of either delirium tremens or withdrawal seizures. The clinician should monitor the patient's withdrawal symptoms and vital signs and be proactive in referring the patient for qualified medical assessment and medical clearance by an emergency department.

Benzodiazepines

Like alcohol, benzodiazepines also depress the central nervous system and are mostly prescribed for anxiety symptoms.[16] This drug class includes Valium, Xanax, Ativan, and Klonopin. Clinically, benzodiazepines are intended to be used temporarily, but there is a prevalence of extended use that leads to tolerance and dependence. Like alcohol, tolerance means requiring more to relieve anxiety and prevent withdrawal. Many dependent individuals abuse or overuse their prescriptions and illicitly obtain them until the next prescription can be filled.[17] The effects of benzodiazepine abuse are like alcohol with respect to slowed cognitive processing, euphoria, relaxed state, and impaired motor skills.

The withdrawal symptoms from benzodiazepines are like that of alcohol withdrawal in terms of anxiety, irritability, shaking, headache, nausea/vomiting, and body aches. Foremost of concern is the risk for withdrawal seizures. Again, the clinician should screen for patient history of withdrawal seizures or seizures in general.[18] The clinician should closely monitor the patients' withdrawal symptoms during the interview.

Alcohol and benzodiazepine detox are measured by the Clinical Institute Withdrawal Assessment (CIWA) scale (table 8.2). Withdrawal from these substances is potentially lethal. The three indicators for potentially severe or lethal withdrawal from alcohol or benzodiazepines include

- a CIWA score of fifteen or higher,
- a history of withdrawal seizures or delirium tremens, and
- daily consumption of a "significant amount" of benzodiazepines.[19]

A scenario of this significant amount is a patient reporting daily use of eight milligrams of Xanax per day even if they are not experiencing withdrawal and deny a history of withdrawal seizures or delirium tremens.

Like the COWS, the information for the CIWA is gathered by observing for the categories of symptoms and asking the patient questions. The last section of the CIWA involves orientation that includes asking a patient "serial additions." In this last section, if the patient missed the day or date by more than two days, the patient scores a "2." However, there is challenge of asking patients to do "serial additions" when they correctly name the current date. An example of serial additions is: "Can you add threes up to the number thirty?"

It may be just effective to borrow from the mini-mental-status examination and ask the patient to do serial subtractions such as counting backwards from twenty by threes or backwards from one hundred by sevens. Examples of these questions are as follows:

Table 8.2. Clinical Institute Withdrawal Assessment of Alcohol Scale, Revised

Pulse: ____________________ Blood Pressure: ____________

NAUSEA AND VOMITIING: Ask *"Do you feel sick to your stomach? Have you vomited?"* Observation: 0 No nausea and no vomiting 1 Mild nausea and no vomiting 2 3 4 Intermittent nausea with dry heaves 5 6 7 Constant nausea, frequent dry heaves, and vomiting	**AUDITORY DISTURBANCES:** Ask *"Are you more aware of sounds around you? Are they harsh? Do they frighten you? Are you hearing anything that is disturbing to you? Are you hearing things you know are not there?"* Observation: 0 Not present 1 Very mild harshness or ability to frighten 2 Mild harness or ability to frighten 3 Moderate harshness or ability to frighten 4 Moderately severe hallucinations 5 Severe hallucinations 6 Extremely severe hallucinations 7 Continuous hallucinations
TREMOR: Arms extended and fingers spread apart. Observation: 0 No tremor 1 Not visible, but can be felt fingertip to fingertip 2 3 4 Moderate, with patient's arms extended 5 6 7 Severe, even with arms not extended	**VISUAL HALLUCINATIONS:** Ask *"Does the light appear to be too bright? Is its color different? Does it hurt your eyes? Are you seeing anything that is disturbing to you? Are you seeing things you know are not there?"* Observation: 0 Not present 1 Very mild sensitivity 2 Mild sensitivity 3 Moderate sensitivity 4 Moderately severe hallucinations 5 Severe hallucinations 6 Extremely severe hallucinations 7 Continuous hallucinations
PAROXYSMAL SWEATS: Observation: 0 No sweat visible 1 Barely perceptible sweating, palms moist 2 3 4 Beads of sweat obvious on forehead 5 6 7 Drenching sweats	**HEADACHE, FULLNESS IN HEAD:** Ask *"Does your head feel different? Does it feel like there is a band around your head?"* Do not rate for dizziness or lightheadedness. Otherwise, rate severity. 0 Not present 1 Very mild 2 Mild 3 Moderate 4 Moderately severe 5 Severe 6 Very severe 7 Extremely severe

(*Continued*)

Table 8.2. (Continued)

ANXIETY: Ask *"Do you feel nervous?"* Observation: 0 No anxiety, at ease 1 Mild anxiety 2 3 4 Moderately anxious, or guarded so anxiety is inferred 5 6 7 Equivalent to panic states	**ORIENTATION AND CLOUDING OF SENSORIUM:** Ask *"What day is this? Where are you? Who am I?"* 0 Oriented and can do "serial additions" 1 Cannot do serial additions or is uncertain about date 2 Disoriented for date by no more than two calendar dates 3 Disoriented for date by more than two calendar dates 4 Disoriented for place/or person
AGITATION: Observation: 0 Normal activity 1 Somewhat more than normal activity 2 3 4 Moderately fidgety and restless 5 6 7 Paces back and forth during most of the interview, or constantly thrashes about	**Blood Pressure:** 0 Less than 140/90 1 140/90–150/98 2 160/100–175/110 3 176/110–199/110 4 More than 200/110
TACTILE DISTURBANCES: Ask *"Have you any itching, pins and needles sensations, burning, numbness, or do you feel bugs crawling on or under your skin?"* Observation: 0 None 1 Very mild itching, pins and needles, burning, or numbness 2 Mild itching, pins and needles, burning, or numbness 3 Moderate itching, pins and needles, burning, or numbness 4 Moderately severe hallucinations 5 Severe hallucinations 6 Extremely severe hallucinations 7 Continuous hallucinations	**Pulse:** 0 90 or less 1 91–100 2 101–120 3 121–139 4 140 or more
	Total Points: ________________

Note: From J. T. Sullivan, K. Sykora, J. Schneiderman, C. A. Naranjo, and E. M. Sellers, 1989, "Assessment of alcohol withdrawal: The revised Clinical Institute Withdrawal Assessment for Alcohol scale (CIWA-Ar)," *British Journal of Addiction, 84*(11): 1353–57.

- Can you count backwards from one hundred by sevens? Instead of going one hundred, ninety-nine, ninety-eight, ninety-seven, etc., can you start at one hundred and count down by sevens?[20]
- Can you count backwards from twenty by threes? Instead of going twenty, nineteen, eighteen, seventeen, etc., start at twenty and count down by threes.[21]

Stop the patient after five answers. Some patients may automatically say that they cannot do this. If the patient gets it wrong or refuses to do it, they would be given a score of "2" for this CIWA category.

Lastly when it comes to the CIWA (and the COWS) is the matter of the patient's vital signs. Both the blood pressure and pulse should have some congruence with the rest of the patient's reported physical symptoms. Part of job orientation should be training on taking vital signs. If clinicians are not trained on taking vital signs, there should be a technician or nurse available to provide this information. If it is a telehealth situation where the patient is at an emergency room, the clinician should get the vitals from emergency department staff in the collateral information prior to the interview.

CRITERIA FOR HOSPITAL ADMISSION

This book has subscribed to "InterQual"[22] as the reference set of admission criteria in determining the level of care. It is indeed a widely accepted standard when it comes to substance use and detox. However, the ASAM criteria has also emerged as a standard. Insurance carriers and managed care companies will often specify which criteria is to be used when conducting prior authorization (see chapter 12). Depending on the setting, the assessment clinician may not be required to master the applications of InterQual or ASAM criteria to begin conducting assessments and making treatment recommendations, but mindfulness of these standards is necessary both when interviewing patients and talking with insurance reviewers using InterQual or ASAM terms or jargon.

As highlighted earlier, InterQual is essentially a published, proprietary collection of criteria used by various managed care organizations for utilization in decision-making. It had been a series of paper manuals and is now online. Access to InterQual is dependent on an organization's willingness to subscribe and acquire the current version. The managed care organization may use it without mention to the hospital. Historically, InterQual can be understood as a continuum of symptom severity and functional impairment for each category of clinical situation. It has spelled out the scenarios for when a patient meets criteria for the different levels of care along the continuum. For the assessment clinician, the important dividing line in InterQual has been immediate safety risk versus potential safety risk.

IMMEDIATE SAFETY RISK VERSUS POTENTIAL SAFETY RISK

As discussed earlier in the book, an immediate safety risk is where the patient is a physical danger to self and/or others due to the collection of observed symptoms and required level of care. The potential safety risk suggests that there may be the need for inpatient admission, but it is dependent on the level of functional impairment (severe, moderate, mild).

The immediate safety risk in InterQual is an objective CIWA score of fifteen,[23] or objectively observable physical symptoms due to alcohol/benzodiazepine withdrawal. The COWS scale discussed earlier was not cited in the InterQual criteria versions available to the authors, but a serious safety risk tends to exist when the patient reports going through opioid withdrawal and evidences a score in the moderate range (twelve to twenty-four).

The ASAM criteria, which is widely available online, has six dimensions of assessment where each dimension represents a level of risk. The dimensions are collections of objective guidelines that suggest the appropriate level of care based on patient presentation. These dimensions are as follows:

- Dimension #1: Acute intoxication and/or withdrawal potential
- Dimension #2: Biomedical conditions and complications
- Dimension #3: Emotional, behavioral, or cognitive conditions and complications
- Dimension #4: Readiness to change
- Dimension #5: Relapse, continued use, or continued problem potential
- Dimension #6: Recovery and living environment

The assessment clinician using ASAM will then apply ordinal ratings to each dimension: none, mild, moderate, and high. There are numerical values of zero to four that correspond to the ordinal ratings.

There is a sense of irony to the ASAM criteria. A patient will logically score high ASAM ratings as follows:

- Dimension #1: The patient is highly intoxicated, has a CIWA of fifteen, a COWS of twelve, or history of complicated detox
- Dimension #2: The patient has severe symptoms of high pulse or pressure, or detox seizures
- Dimension #3: The patient reports suicidal ideations, homicidal ideations, or is psychotic

- Dimension #5: The patient has a history of multiple relapses and makes no statement of needing to stop
- Dimension #6: The patient makes no statement of being connected to sober support and has not been going to support meetings

If a patient demonstrates or verbalizes desire to change, they would get a "low" rating in dimension #4.[24] Otherwise, the rest of the ASAM dimensions lean toward a logical high score to denote severity.

Assigning corresponding numerical scores to the ASAM dimensions will likely be done by the insurance reviewer. Otherwise, it serves to note the ASAM level of care recommendations based on the assessment are as follows:

- Early intervention/driving under the influence program (Level 0.5): Dimensions 1, 2, 3, and 4 stable. Dimensions 5 and 6 are potentially problematic.
- Outpatient treatment (Level 1.0): Dimensions 1, 2, 3, 5, and 6 only mild problems. Dimension 4 is problematic.
- Intensive outpatient treatment (Level 2.1): Dimensions 1 and 2 stable. Dimension 3 mild severity. Dimensions 4, 5, and 6 mild to moderate severity.
- Partial hospital program (Level 2.5): Dimensions 1, 2, and 3 warrant daily monitoring or management. Meet moderate severity in two out of three of Dimensions 4, 5, or 6.
- Residential treatment (Level 3.1—e.g., halfway house): Problems in Dimensions 5 and 6.
- Residential treatment (Level 3.3—e.g., extended/long-term care): Mild to moderate severity in Dimension 3 and in two out of three of Dimensions 4, 5, or 6. Not used for adolescents.
- Residential treatment (Level 3.5): Significant problems in Dimensions 3 and 6; moderate problems in Dimensions 4 and 5.
- Residential treatment (Level 3.7): Functional deficits in two out of three of Dimensions 1, 2, or 3; moderate severity in Dimensions 4, 5, and 6.
- Inpatient treatment (Level 4.0): Severe problems in Dimensions 1, 2, or 3. Problems in the other dimensions do not qualify for this level of care.

The assessment interview results should easily provide answers as to whether the patient is going to meet level 4.0, which should be the following:

- A CIWA of fifteen when the patient seeks detox from alcohol or benzodiazepines
- A history of complicated withdrawal (seizures and delirium tremens)
- Prolonged usage (daily heavy use for at least last consecutive two weeks) and intoxication
- A COWS of twelve or higher.

Clarifications

Beyond the ASAM and InterQual criteria, it is important to note that patients detoxing from the following substances do not qualify for inpatient detox in and of themselves:

1. Cannabis
2. Stimulants (cocaine/amphetamines)
3. Synthetic drugs
4. Psychedelics

If a patient is going to meet criteria for inpatient admission seeking detox from this latter set of substances, there must be some co-morbid suicidal ideation or severe psychosis that constitutes an immediate safety risk and would get a high rating on Dimension #3; however, the primary diagnosis for insurance purposes would be primarily psychiatric and not substance use.

Furthermore, in the matter of dual diagnosis or co-morbidity, many patients who present as psychotic and aggressive may have substance-induced psychosis. In terms of the curve of ability discussed in chapter 2, their impairment may be so great that they are cognitively and behaviorally unable to take part in the interview.

It may not be evident what caused the psychosis until after the patient has been admitted and discloses the substance use. The matter of admissions for substance-induced psychosis is often repetitive, and the clinician or assessment team can get prior experience with the patient, the patient's previous behavior, and the patient's use patterns. With these repetitive patients with known substance use history, a conclusion can reasonably be drawn that the psychosis is substance induced in subsequent presentations; however, the patient should be admitted under a primary psychiatric and not a mental health diagnosis.

Detox and obvious psychosis aside, the patient who is intoxicated and reporting suicidal ideation without a plan, homicidal ideation without a plan, or command hallucinations is considered an immediate safety risk. Intoxication increases the risk of danger to self or others given the increased tendency of impulsivity and mood fluctuation.

Referrals to Other Levels of Care

A patient who is not evidencing an immediate safety risk nor sufficient functional impairment to be admitted may meet criteria to go to a residential setting or the partial or intensive outpatient program levels of care. The patient may also evidence some symptoms of detox that are not meeting criteria for inpatient admission. The ASAM level of care recommendations discussed previously can be of help in discerning whether a patient is meeting criteria for residential treatment versus going to a partial or intensive outpatient treatment.

The patient meeting the criteria for these lower levels of care have some kind of impairment in their daily functioning and/or have been referred to treatment by an employer or legal authority. The patient may have to adhere to some stipulations or requirements imposed on them to maintain their employment or avoid further legal consequences. The patient may present with a statement of clear expectations to be in residential treatment and not meet criteria for even that level of care, for which the clinician may have to provide a "note" stating that fact. However, insurance and managed care organizations readily tend to pay for the substance use partial and intensive outpatient when the patient is referred as a condition of employment, probation, or parole.

CONCLUDING THOUGHTS

Substance use assessments can be a very gratifying and fulfilling experience for the assessment clinician. The clinician has the opportunity to be part of a potential lifesaving change for many patients! However, there may be some initial trepidation in conducting the interview given that substance use treatment is a clinical specialty.

Nevertheless, the assessment clinician will get practice in asking substance use questions because they are part of the standard assessment; every patient is going to be screened for substance use. However, the significance of these questions varies depending on the patient's presenting problems and complaints. They ironically become more difficult when the patient is presenting for substance use issues.

Motivation for treatment is often an emotional matter for the patient. The patient's motivation may be out of anger when compelled by an authority or out of fear when thinking about the pain of detox. It is our experience that addicted people are fragile when they truly come forward and talk about how much they used and how often they have used. It serves to repeat from chapter 4 that if there is a trauma history that is reviewed prior to the substance use questions, there may be significant transference and avoidance on the patient's part to give factual answers.

The learning curve in substance use assessment is repetitively experiencing the presentation of detox and intoxication and managing the roadblocks that the patient puts up in answering the questions. Regardless of the patient's roadblocks, the clinician must conclude whether criteria for admission have been met to a particular level of care. However, above determining if criteria have been met, the medical danger of drug use must be recognized and the clinician is further challenged to assess for medical risk.

Lastly, as a matter of foreshadowing, not everyone is going to meet criteria for admission to the hospital for detox. The clinician sadly must be the doorkeeper in assertively telling a patient that they do not meet criteria for admission. We discuss this challenge in chapter 11.

However, there will be some patients not meeting criteria for detox admission who are highly motivated to get into the hospital no matter the reason and will then say they are suicidal with a plan, which makes the admission a psychiatric one. It is a challenge not to be in an emotional power struggle with such patients. As professionals, our job is establishing whether the facts exist to demonstrate that criteria is met and not keeping patients out of the hospital.

NOTES

1. There are distinct criteria between the partial hospitalization and intensive outpatient levels of care based on symptom severity. However, some payor sources will not pay partial hospitalization but will pay for intensive outpatient. On the other hand, some other payor sources (particularly managed Medicare) will not pay for intensive outpatient but will pay for partial hospitalization. Furthermore, there are hospital preferences to bill solely at the intensive outpatient level which determine what is offered to patients. For more information on these levels of care, see D. Houvenagle, 2015, *Clinician's guide to partial hospitalization and intensive outpatient practice*, New York: Springer.
2. There are psychiatric hospitals that offer the residential level of care and sober living as follow-up treatment.
3. Having an appreciation of the stages of change can be helpful in understanding why some substance use patients come for detox and then leave either before assessment or actual admission to the unit. J. O. Prochaska and J. C. Norcross, 2001, "Stages of change," *Psychotherapy: Theory, Research, Practice, Training, 38*(4): 443–48.
4. An embarrassed patient may be exhibiting multiple negative cognitions that include mind reading that the clinician is judging them.
5. While not discussed in detail here, there are two common scenarios of exaggeration. One situation is typically by a high utilizer who will simultaneously report high use or detox with psychiatric symptoms (suicidal with a specific plan or psychosis). The second scenario is when couples come in together to detox. One partner likely has authentic symptoms that meet inpatient criteria while the other must exaggerate symptoms to get admitted. There are "couple" scenarios where one exaggerated detox symptoms to meet criteria and the other was not admitted, and the exaggerating patient then demanded to leave and declined admission. The reality of exaggeration in detox symptoms can include that some patients can be excellent actors to achieve admission.

6. The easiest technique for fostering a safe place is the use of the "modified boredom" technique. The clinician may also have to make statements of empathy such as "I am not here to judge you but help you get the help you are seeking."

7. If the patient is being seen an emergency department, it is expected that the patient has been medically cleared prior to the clinician being called for the assessment.

8. These are trade names for amphetamine, dextroamphetamine mixed salts, methylphenidate ER, and Methylphenidate hydrochloride.

9. There is a product called "Delta-8 tetrahydrocannabinol" that is a derivative of hemp that can give the user the same effect as using marijuana. It can show up in drug screens as a cannabinoid. At the time of writing, it is not illegal to sell in multiple states, and it is available in retail stores.

10. D. R. Wesson and W. Ling, 2003, "The clinical opiate withdrawal scale (COWS)," *Journal of Psychoactive Drugs, 35*(2): 253–59.

11. This is an author suggestion versus an actual prescribed question on the COWS.

12. For many opioid users, there is a narrow window of motivation to come in and detox. There is a social learning process where word gets passed around that to get admitted before severe detox symptoms occur one must say that they are suicidal. Of course, this is lying, and such patients will only admit that "I just said that to get admitted" to inpatient staff when conducting follow-up assessments for suicidal ideation. There is a high likelihood that a patient not getting admitted will go back out and use to avoid detox.

13. Malt liquor is essentially a beer that has been brewed in a manner that boosts the alcohol content. Fortified wines have a boosted alcohol content by the addition of brandy or other type of alcohol.

14. It may be a local culture to drink non-potable forms of alcohol. The writers are familiar with the fact that some Native American/First Nations groups have a historical preference of consuming aerosol household disinfectant over potable forms.

15. Highly intoxicated individuals may be unable to blow on a breathalyzer, which may necessitate transport to an emergency department for medical clearance.

16. Benzodiazepines may also be used to treat seizures in medical emergencies. They are used in some detox protocols to prevent seizures. They are also prescribed in cases of catatonia.

17. Many individuals with certain personality disorders fall into this category, as they have problems managing their anxiety through psychotherapy and internalization of coping skills. Because of the tendency for dependence, there has been a trend since the first decade of the 2000s to reduce the number of benzodiazepine prescriptions in favor of alternatives that include hydroxyzine.

18. This should be a standard question on a structured interview.

19. This is at the discretion of the physician.

20. The correct answer is "one hundred, ninety-three, eighty-six, seventy-nine, seventy-two, sixty-five."

21. The correct answer is "twenty, seventeen, fourteen, eleven, eight, five, two."

22. InterQual was previous owned by McKesson Healthcare and at the time of publication is now owned by Change Healthcare, a subsidiary of Optum. There is not

a precise bibliographic reference of the most current form that can be given other than InterQual® | Change Healthcare. https://www.changehealthcare.com/solutions/interqual.

23. Also, at the physician's discretion in accordance with InterQual, a patient could have a CIWA score of eight to fourteen and potentially be admitted if they have a pulse greater than or equal to one hundred or if their blood pressure is greater than or equal to 150/90. A physician can also consider admitting an individual based on "withdrawal syndrome" in which they have experienced any of the following: a seizure, protracted vomiting, postural systolic BP drop of greater than thirty, a temperature greater than 101 degrees Fahrenheit, a pulse greater than or equal to 120 beats per minute, a blood pressure greater than or equal to 160/100, or disorientation to place or person.

24. An example of a patient scoring a mild or higher on ASAM Dimension #4 is as follows. A male with repeated admissions who has significant personality disorder features and regularly high blood alcohol levels comes in saying that they need to detox. However, part of the collateral information or interview itself is that while intoxicated the patient stated suicidal ideation with one or more lethal plans. Such a patient avoids a statement that they need to stop using.

Chapter 9

Language Interpretation

Behavioral health crisis knows no language. Many who have come to North America for the safety and economic opportunity did not expect themselves nor their family members to have mental health crises. However, crises do happen, and the typical assessment clinician will have to interview patients requiring a language interpreter. On the other hand, individuals who are deaf will also come for themselves or with their family members and will also require an interpreter. Besides the essential decency of using an interpreter, it is required by law under Title VI of the 1964 Civil Rights Act and other federal regulations.

Besides the law, there are ethical considerations that include the respect for the self-determination of the patient. In the North American and European contexts, the patient, regardless of age, gender, or previous culture, has rights to privacy, self-determination, and professional competency in the assessment. Family members can offer to translate but stigma, embarrassment, family dynamics, and lack of knowledge of medical terminology can all interfere with the patient's rights and end in professional liability for the clinician and the organization. A qualified, impartial interpreter is a must.

Becoming accustomed to working with an interpreter is a development process. While the interpreter is technically a third party in the encounter, *they are not another person in the conversation.* The interpreter provides the impartial service as the voice of the clinician and the confidential voice of the patient, nothing more and nothing less. The clinician should talk directly to the patient as if conducting a conversation in the clinician's native language. It is initially awkward, but with practice the clinician should come across as having a normal interview.

The requirement of the interpreter extends the length of the interview. It is a simple logic of more words equaling more time. The interview can take even longer, depending on the cognitive impairment of the patient due to psychosis or intoxication.

Even with getting accustomed to using an interpreter, there will still be challenging if not tricky clinical situations that include telehealth and child-adolescent interviews. The telehealth interviews will involve both the video link and simultaneous telephone conversation. The child-adolescent interviews typically involve a child fluent in English and a parent who speaks little English or is deaf. The language disparity between the child and parent also can equal a power struggle or imbalance that can result in arguments in another language that extends the interview further and leaves the clinician struggling to capture all the salient information.

This chapter discusses considerations and techniques for using interpreters in assessment interviews. It will discuss the legal and ethical imperatives and then techniques and approaches for using interpreters.

LEGAL AND ETHICAL CONSIDERATIONS

The legal and ethical responsibilities of managing professional language interpretation comes down to using only licensed or certified language interpreters to interview patients; otherwise, the hospital or healthcare setting can be liable for malpractice.[1] Hadziabdic and Hjelm (2013) noted that "When a person is not able to communicate or lacks words or expressions for his or her needs and desires there is an obvious risk of misdiagnosis which can lead to inappropriate treatment."[2] On the level of basic decency, Napoles et al. (2015) found that patients with limited English proficiency had poorer outcomes when untrained interpreters were used due to "inaccurate language interpretation."[3] Patients not only deserve access to quality and accurate healthcare in accordance with their rights but again on the legal front may have recourse for inappropriate interpretation completed by someone without the proper training.

Family and friends should not interpret for the patient due to concerns for confounding variables such as privacy, impartiality, and accuracy. A patient might not want their sibling who is translating to know certain personal information and therefore withhold it in the interview. Or the sibling who is translating may disagree with the patient's statements and "translate" inaccurately. A domestic violence situation or manipulative dynamic also can be masked when a potential abuser is translating for the patient.

Furthermore, a hospital employee might speak the patient's native tongue or know sign language, but they should not interpret unless they are a certified interpreter. Just speaking the same language does not mean that the employee can validly and accurately interpret medical terms and represent cultural context. If an adverse event occurs when a hospital employee is used as a non-certified interpreter, the hospital and clinician are open to liability. A certified medical language interpreter has been tested as to knowledge of relevant terminology and the competency of ability to interpret at a certain pace for an extended length of time.

What is more, interpreters should be expected to be detached professionals with commensurate standards. They are solely there to translate between the patient and clinician in a confidential manner. They are not there to socialize with the patient or family, and any in-person interpreter should wait in nursing stations.[4] At the beginning of the interview, the interpreter should introduce themselves to the patient and give a preamble that the interview is confidential.

To comply with legal and ethical imperatives, the typical hospital contracts with one or more interpreter services that range from in-person to video teleconferencing/telehealth to phone. Resource availability is dependent upon the population, size of the local area, and organizational budget. If within a locality where there is a high density of a particular language group with a high utilization rate, then there will likely be onsite, qualified, face-to-face interpreters who are either contracted or directly employed by hospitals. With the improvement of internet and data signals and installation of Wi-Fi in hospitals, video interpreter service is increasingly available; otherwise, the clinician will have access to translators over the phone.

To access the service, the clinician must give identifying information of some form for billing purposes. The information can vary from simply the unit name/number and the clinician's name to patient record numbers. The hospital in which the clinician is doing the assessment should be providing the service and the appropriate access credentials to the clinician.

The phone interpretation options depend on the hardware available, the modernity of the facility, and building layout. A special phone may be offered by interpretation services where the clinician and the patient have handsets to be on the line simultaneously. While it is less than optimal, the clinician may have to settle for a speaker landline phone. While it is not encouraged, some clinicians may have to use a personal mobile phone and its speaker option when no other working hardware is to be found. This is particularly challenging depending on the ambient noise of the physical setting and the number of people involved in the interview.

The interpreter service itself can be limited in options. Interpreters can be in high demand in the morning hours when healthcare organizations have full clinic and testing schedules. Some languages are rarer than others. Furthermore, some dialects are not available at all, and the interpreter service may ask if the patient speaks a different language.

In cases where the interpreter service cannot provide an interpreter, and it appears to be imperative to use a family member or hospital employee, the clinician should document the attempts to secure the services of a qualified interpreter. The documentation should be precise in terms of the language, exact times of attempts and the response of the interpreter service about unavailability, and the inability of the patient to speak another language. The purpose of such documentation is to mitigate liability and demonstrate effort to respect the patient's rights.

Regardless, documentation is essential in interpretation situations to establish that the rights of the patient were upheld and maintained. The clinician should document the name of the service, the interpreter identification number, and the language of the patient.

EXPECTATIONS FOR THE INTERVIEW

Conducting an interview through an interpreter can be scary the first time, and maybe the apprehension will return the first time the clinician gets a different language. There is fear of inaccurately assessing the problem and offending the patient. Then there are the pressures of time. However, the clinician should expect the same logic in answers as if conducting an interview with a native English-speaking person with a few challenges.

The primary challenge is if the patient is impaired. Such impairment could be psychosis with disorganized thinking. An intoxicated or severely detoxing patient may be half asleep and slow to answer the questions. The patient's answers through the interpreter may be illogical, and the interpreter may comment on the patient's problems of answering.

The other challenges include the English fluency of the interpreter, quality of the mode (video/phone), and environmental/background noise. While a professional interpreter is sufficiently fluent in both languages to meet a certain accreditation standard, some interpreters have heavy accents that require the clinician to ask for ongoing repetition for clarity in patient response. A bad telephone line by itself further complicates matters, especially if the interpreter has a heavy accent. The interview will have to go at a slower pace, and the clinician must demonstrate patience to ensure accurate history taking.

There is the risk of increased confusion and chaos when there are family members present with the patient in the interview who also need interpretation. The patient and family members may argue with each other in their own language which the interpreter cannot fully translate and thus the clinician will not fully understand. Therefore, a good principle for managing such situations is interviewing one person at a time. While it further lengthens the time required for the interview, it is orderly, and the clinician is more likely to be able to collect all relevant collateral from the family in a calm fashion. However, the emotional needs of the family may have to be attended to at the beginning of the interview by way of an empathetic introduction and an explanation of how the clinician will conduct the interview with the patient and them. An example of this interpretation situation will be illustrated in the vignettes.

TELEHEALTH

The global COVID-19 outbreak made telehealth a necessity as a socially distanced manner of service delivery, but prior to the epidemic, it had been increasingly used in providing mental health assessment to multiple emergency rooms and other acceptable sites in an efficient manner.[5] With telehealth, one clinician can remain stationary and perform assessments for multiple, linked sites within the same state. Telehealth interviewing itself without language interpretation presents numerous challenges. These challenges include

- quality of the online link/signal,
- connection of the interpreter into the online meeting,
- quality of the computer hardware used by the telehealth location,
- background noise at the patient's telehealth location (emergency department chatter),
- medical acuity of the patient,
- inability to observe body language and facial expressions readily observable in an in-person assessment due to the computer,
- risk of less patient engagement related to cultural attitudes of being interviewed over telehealth,
- interviewing family members present, and
- assessing physical symptoms of detox (tremors, diaphoresis, eye pupil dilation).

These challenges are different forms of interference in the communication process between the patient and clinician that can be frustrating even if talking to one person at a time. The computer hardware at the patient's site may be a tablet computer with poor bandwidth or a marginal camera and a marginal microphone that provides a small picture and picks up the background noise more than the patient's soft voice.

The best option for telehealth with an interpreter is to have the interpreter logged into the same video conferencing room or meeting. Otherwise, the second-best option is having patient on the video link and have the interpreter over the phone. The clinician can see the patient over the video link and talk through the interpreter via the phone line. When the phone line must be used, it increases the likelihood of keeping the patient's attention and it can compensate for the telehealth link limitations.

Another way to compensate for the awkwardness of the telehealth situation is empathetic recognition. The clinician's use of paraverbal communication that includes empathy can help influence the patient to participate in a more active manner. It can help for the clinician to make a statement that intentionally recognizes the patient's humanity and the uniqueness of this situation. An example is: "Ms. _____, sorry for the awkwardness of this situation, but it is going to be thc best way to do this interview." This kind of approach requires mindfulness on the part of the clinician.

VIGNETTES

The following are vignettes demonstrating using an interpreter. They start with the interaction with the interpreter. Such vignettes are of limited value in this chapter because they would only be in English like other vignettes in this book.

Vignette #1: A Basic Interview with an Interpreter

Eduardo Gonzalez is thirty-eight-year-old male who presented for assessment. The registration clerk had identified that Mr. Gonzalez had limited English language skills and notified the clinician that Mr. Gonzalez would need an interpreter. The clinician set up the interpretation phone set in the interview room, called Mr. Gonzalez in, and dialed the number to the interview service. The vignette started when the interpreter answered the phone.

Interpreter: Hello, my name is Jose, Spanish language interpreter #228932. What unit are you calling from?

Clinician: Good morning, Jose. My name is John, and I work in the Oak Leaf Hospital Admitting Department. I am in need of interpretation services for an assessment interview.

Interpreter: I'd be glad to help. What is the patient's identification number?

Clinician: The identification number is 3544354543.

Interpreter: Very good sir. Is the patient with you?

Clinician: Yes, he is.

Interpreter: May I introduce myself?

Clinician: Please go ahead.

Interpreter: *A statement of purpose and confidentiality in Spanish, and then said in English:* I am ready for your instruction.

Clinician: Jose, I will try to keep my sentences short, and I will say "Go ahead" to cue you to interpret.

Interpreter: Very good sir.

Clinician: Good morning, Mr. Gonzalez. My name is John, and I am an assessment clinician here at Oak Leaf Hospital. I have been here ten years. This a confidential interview with two exceptions. If someone reports abuse, I may have to report it to protective services, and if someone reports having thoughts of wanting to hurt or kill another person, I have a duty to warn. Otherwise, what is said here stays here. Go ahead.

Interpreter: *(translates/interprets for patient)*

Patient: *(responds in primary language)*

Interpreter: *(translate/interprets for clinician)* Okay.

Clinician: Mr. Gonzalez, what brings you in to talk to us today? Go ahead.

Interpreter: *(translates/interprets for patient)*

Patient: *(responds in primary language)*

Interpreter: *(translate/interprets for clinician)*

The interview continued without incident. Mr. Gonzalez reported that he had been having suicidal thoughts. He was offered inpatient admission and accepted the treatment recommendation.

Vignette #2: When Family Is Present

Maria Fernandez is a fifty-five-year-old female who presented with her daughter. Her daughter immediately started speaking.

Daughter: Hello, my mother does not speak English. I am here to interpret for her.

Clinician: I am glad that you are willing to do that for your mother. However, we are legally required to use certified medical interpreters.

Daughter: Will it cost us money for the interpreter?

Clinician: No. The hospital is required to pay for the interpreter. It will not cost you anything. I will be right back with the interpreter tablet (computer).

The clinician went to the office and got the tablet computer. He logged on and was able to get a videocall with a Spanish language interpreter. He commenced with the interview.

Interpreter: This is Josue, Spanish interpreter number #295678. I will be your interpreter. What is the name of the unit?

Clinician: Admitting.

Interpreter: And what is your name?

Clinician: David Smith.

Interpreter: Very good. Is the patient with you?

Clinician: Yes.

Interpreter: May I introduce myself?

Clinician: Yes *(turns the screen to the patient).*

Interpreter: *(introduced self in Spanish, gives disclaimer that the conversation is confidential then said in English)* I am now ready for your instruction.

Clinician: Ms. Fernandez, my name is David. I am assessment clinician. I have been with the hospital for fifteen years. This is a confidential interview. The questions are on my screen. I will type your answers into the computer. The interview will hopefully take no more than one hour. What said here will stay here. The exceptions to confidentiality are if someone reports abuse and neglect or if someone reports wanting to hurt or kill another person. Go ahead. *(clinician pauses for the interpreter)*

WORKING WITH THE INTERPRETER

The following are some suggested guidelines for working with an interpreter:

- Speak in complete thoughts.
- Speak in short sentences.
- Talk in a normal speaking voice and volume.
- Tell the interpreter the nature of the interview at the beginning.
- Tell the interpreter that you will use the cue "go ahead" when you are wanting them to translate.
- Do not say "Tell the patient." Always talk directly to the patient.

CONCLUDING THOUGHTS

Using a qualified interpreter is a legal and ethical imperative. No matter what language a patient speaks, they are entitled to impartial and confidential language translation. The frequency of using translation services depends on the population density of people with limited English skills in a local area.

In the twenty-first century, technological advancement has allowed more access to interpretation services by audio or video. However, such technology is imperfect and subject to interference distortion both by signal weakness and background noise. Nevertheless, it saves time over waiting hours for an interpreter to arrive and be present to translate.

There can be a sense of angst when the next patient is one who needs an interpreter for themselves or a family member. Yes, it will take more time and there is always the mystery of how good the English language skills of the interpreter will be. However, imagine you, yourself, are stuck in another country where you do not speak the language and you or a family member are having some kind of emergency.

Your angst might be ramped up a few notches. You do not know the system. You do not know whether the professionals will be receptive or respectful to you. You do not know whether there is an interpreter that will get it right and you or your family member will get what you need.

This last vignette is meant to be a journey in empathy and perhaps an attitude adjustment. Assessment clinicians are the trusted individuals in society in place to help vulnerable people in crisis regardless of language spoken. There has been too much of a history where immigrants who have no or limited language skills have been exploited, abused, and neglected by perpetrators of opportunity. For the assessment clinician, every patient and their family members are people with worth and dignity. There will also be the temptation to think "Not another one of these . . . I am too tired," but as professionals we must find it within ourselves to manage our attitudes and do what is right because it is the right thing.

NOTES

1. K. Quan, 2011, "The high costs of language barriers in medical malpractice," National Law Program Berkley CA, University of California–Berkley. This report consists of cases of malpractice settlements where there was inappropriate communication with non-English speakers and there were bad outcomes.

2. E. Hadziabdic and K. Hjelm, 2013, "Working with interpreters: Practical advice for use of an interpreter in healthcare," *International Journal of Evidence-Based Healthcare, 11*: 69–76.

3. A. M. Nápoles, J. Santoyo-Olsson, L. S. Karliner, S. E. Gregorich, and E. J. Pérez-Stable, 2015, "Inaccurate language interpretation and its clinical significance in the medical encounters of Spanish-speaking Latinos," *Medical Care, 53*(11): 940–47.

4. This is especially crucial when the patient and family are being argumentative. The interpreter may know the language but that does not give them license to get involved in the conflict. Getting involved in the conflict destroys the impartiality and integrity of accurate interpretation.

5. It is the opinion of the authors that telehealth assessment interviews should only be done with emergency room sites or other secure sites such as a residential treatment facility. Telehealth assessments should not be done with patients in their homes in the name of confidentiality and safety.

Chapter 10

Staffing with the Doctors

The next step after finishing the interview is staffing the patient's case with a relevant psychiatrist or psychiatric nurse practitioner. The doctor or the nurse practitioner is the deciding authority about admission, and the assessment clinician is their eyes and ears on a patient. It is a challenge because the clinician is seeking to condense fifteen minutes to two hours' worth of information into a phone call that is a less than a minute.

Metaphorically, the assessment clinician becomes a broadcast news reporter delivering a live report. The assessment clinician is one of many who call a practitioner at all hours of the night and day and so it may not necessarily be welcome but possibly intrusive versus annoying.[1] A clinician giving unnecessary information can increase the likelihood of expressed annoyance by the practitioner. The practitioner may also be multi-tasking and the assessment clinician's call is just another item competing for attention. Therefore, the assessment clinician must both concisely and precisely tell the practitioner the salient facts of the case as clearly and audibly as possible while sounding calm, in a business-like fashion.

This reporting process has the potential of being mentally and emotionally draining. The patient interview may have been difficult, stressful, or chaotic due to the subject matter, patient behavior, or family conflict that manifested. The clinician must change gears mentally and move from the emotions of the interview to a rational and factual mindset about whether the patient has met criteria for admission.

As part of job orientation, some hospitals have training that addresses this step. New clinicians may have to first staff the case with a supervisor or senior staff member before going to the doctor or nurse practitioner. However, some job situations do not give this training and the new clinician does this by trial and possibly embarrassing and frustrating error, and it can lead to premature exit from the job that could have been prevented.

This chapter covers skills in staffing cases after the assessment with practitioners. It will discuss suggested scripts, delivery of the scripts, and suggestions for dealing with extraordinary situations. It will close with some typical scenarios demonstrating the techniques.

THE SCRIPT AND ITS ELEMENTS

Essentially a script is a planned, ordered sequence of words and actions. The primary recognized use of a script is in broadcast and theatrical production whether recorded or presented live in front of audiences.[2] However, there are many such scripts that are part of social norms of human interactions (greetings and farewells). The assessment interview indeed is itself an elongated script that has intent and purpose between the clinician and patient. The successful staffing with the practitioner (whether it be a physician or nurse practitioner) should be brief and render a clinical decision whether it be inpatient admission or other recommendation, and the script will be part of it.

THE STRUCTURE OF THE SCRIPT

There are at least seven elements of the staffing script:

- Greeting
- Self-identification of assessment clinician
- Purpose of call
- Identification of patient
- Reason patient presented with a summary of the criteria for or against admission
- Question to practitioner
- Response from practitioner

The summary of the criteria should at most be two to three sentences. The elements can vary in complexity based on the situation and the practitioner, but the scripts will tend to follow this order.

DELIVERY OF THE SCRIPT: TONE AND PACE

The delivery of the script should exude confidence and professionalism on the part of the assessment clinician. The clinician should be delivering the elements clearly, audibly, and calmly with an economy of words. It does require some thought and practice of condensing a sizable amount of data into the few words about the interview results and whether the patient is meeting criteria for admission.

As will be demonstrated in the vignettes, the clinician is essentially telling the practitioner that the patient is or is not meeting criteria for a level of care and the practitioner agrees, disagrees, or passes on the patient. When the practitioner passes on the patient, it does not mean that the patient is not meeting criteria for admission, but the practitioner may not want to admit that type of patient.[3]

GETTING TO KNOW THE DOCTORS YOU WORK WITH

With time and practice, the assessment clinician gets to know the different psychiatrists and nurse practitioners on the particular rotation. The job orientation process hopefully introduces the new clinician to the preferences of the providers, but it is a learning process of repetitively presenting the cases to get expected and appropriate dispositions and clinical decisions with different types of cases. In a grand sense, the assessment clinician develops relationships with each provider in bits and pieces that include an appreciation of how to present a case in various situations and times of day.

The development of the appreciation is helped by most admitting departments maintaining information about insurances, vacations, and rotations. Some providers are not in the network of certain insurances, are on vacation, or are off rotation for various reasons such as caseload size. It is the duty of both the department and the clinician to maintain current awareness of the information.

WHEN A DOCTOR PASSES

There is nothing inherently wrong with the clinician's assessment or presentation if a doctor or provider passes on a patient. The clinician is not a salesperson seeking to persuade but a reporter of a situation. Some doctors have patient preferences and the one just assessed by the clinician may not fit into those profiles. On the other hand, some cases are complicated and a provider may not feel like dealing with it on a given day. Furthermore, a doctor may not want a previous patient again and so they pass. If it is a new patient who has never been previously admitted, the clinician simply goes to the next provider on the rotation.

A doctor passing on a "previous patient" is another matter. The provider may be making a statement and drawing a line that the patient does not need to be admitted. If this is a high utilizer with multiple admissions and who may have just been discharged earlier in the day, the clinician is potentially caught in a paradox.[4] As will be discussed later in the book, the average high utilizer is savvy and will say precisely what is needed to get admitted even it contains provable lies.[5] When this is happening, it is incumbent upon the clinician to talk with a supervisor about the next steps to take in the situation.

THE RISK OF BAD RECOMMENDATIONS

There is the inherent risk of a bad recommendation, especially in the cases of high utilizers, given the clinician's inherent professional liability and vantage point of direct observation. Despite the admission history, inpatient admission may still very well be indicated given the patient's affective presentation. The clinician has several choices in this case that include

- reiterating the patient's affective presentation and assertively suggesting inpatient,
- calling the supervisor to discuss the concerns of the case and obtaining consultation,
- calling the medical director, and
- calling the next provider on the rotation.

The clinician should be an advocate for the patient when the patient presents as needing admission.[6]

EXTRAORDINARY SITUATIONS

There are both routine and extraordinary situations where the clinician must go off a normal script for staffing a case with a provider. There are cases that are "on the line" which do not clearly meet criteria for inpatient admission. Other cases can be confusing. In these situations, the assessment clinician must take more time to lay out the patient details and get a true recommendation or opinion from the practitioner versus agreement that a case does or does not meet criteria for admission. The clinicians will need to tell the provider at the top of the phone call that it is going to take a little more time.

Related to taking more time to staffing the case, there will be extraordinary cases where the clinician may be indecisive over whether to admit or make a recommendation contrary to criteria having been met. There is nothing wrong with asking a provider "what direction should this case go?"

VIGNETTES

This section will demonstrate staffing with practitioners over the phone based on the "InterQual" standards. It assumes that there are rules about "previous patients," where once providers get a patient, they will get that patient in any future admissions. The vignettes will follow this pattern except for the last two examples.

Vignette #1: Adult with Suicidal Ideation

Greeting: Dr. Smith.

Self-identification: This is David at the Memorial Admission Department.

Purpose of call: I am calling you on the inpatient rotation.

Identification of patient: I have a forty-eight-year-old female named Debbie Ryan.

Reason patient presented: She reported being suicidal with a plan today to overdose on a bottle of pills.[7]

Question to practitioner: Would you accept her for admission to inpatient?

Response from practitioner: Yes, I will.

Vignette #2: Adult with Psychosis

Greeting: Dr. Allen.

Self-identification: This is David at the Memorial Admission Department.

Purpose of call: I am calling you on the inpatient rotation.

Identification of patient: I have a twenty-three-year-old male named James Hardin.

Reason patient presented: He reported that he is hearing voices, seeing things, and said that the television is talking specifically about him. He cannot answer the suicide question. I also witnessed him responding to internal stimuli.

Question to practitioner: Would you accept him for admission to inpatient?

Response from practitioner: Yes, I will.

Vignette #3: Adult with Severe Psychosis

Greeting: Dr. Allen.

Self-identification: This is David at the Memorial Admission Department.

Purpose of call: I am calling you on the inpatient rotation.

Identification of patient: I have a thirty-four-year-old male named John Ramsey.

Reason patient presented: He was brought by a neighbor due to bizarre behavior. I observed him responding to internal stimuli and hiding behind the door. He would not respond to any questions including about suicidal ideation or homicidal ideation.

Question to practitioner: Would you admit him on a seventy-two-hour hold?

Response from practitioner: Yes, I will.

Vignette #4: Adult with Alcohol Withdrawal

Greeting: Dr. Wilson.

Self-identification: This is David at the Memorial Admission Department.

Purpose of call: I am calling you on the inpatient rotation.

Identification of patient: I have a thirty-five-year-old female named Wendy Lamke.

Reason patient presented: She is here for detox. She reported that she had been averaging one fifth of liquor per day for the past month. She last consumed about five hours ago. She had a blood alcohol level of 0.12 and a CIWA of fourteen.

Question to practitioner: Would you accept her for admission to inpatient?

Response from practitioner: Yes, I will.

Vignette #5: Adult with Opioid Withdrawal

Greeting: Dr. Sanders.

Self-identification: This is David at the Memorial Admission Department.

Purpose of call: I am calling you on the inpatient rotation.

Identification of patient: I have a thirty-nine-year-old male named Lowell Mooney.

Reason patient presented: He is here requesting opioid detox. He has been using one gram heroin intravenously daily for the past two months with last use today about twelve hours ago. He has a COWS score of fourteen.

Question to practitioner: Would you accept him for admission to inpatient?

Response from practitioner: Yes, I will.

Vignette #6: Adolescent/Child with Suicidal Ideation

Greeting: Dr. Johnson.

Self-identification: This is David at the Memorial Admission Department.

Purpose of call: I am calling you on the child inpatient rotation.

Identification of patient: I have a fifteen-year-old female named Cindy Buehler.

Reason patient presented: She was brought in by her mother and father. She reported that she has been thinking about killing herself with an overdose. She last had the thought this morning.

Question to practitioner: Would you accept her for admission to inpatient?

Response from practitioner: That should be fine.

Vignette #7: Adolescent/Child with Psychosis

Greeting: Dr. Johnson.

Self-identification: This is David at the Memorial Admission Department.

Purpose of call: I am calling you on the child inpatient rotation.

Identification of patient: I have a sixteen-year-old male named Lou Bauer.

Reason patient presented: He was brought in by his mother after a referral from school due to bizarre behavior. The patient also reported that he has been seeing things that make him want to hit others.

Question to practitioner: Would you accept him for admission to inpatient?

Response from practitioner: Yes.

Vignette #8: Child with Out-of-Control Behavior

Greeting: Dr. Johnson.

Self-identification: This is David at the Memorial Admission Department.

Purpose of call: I am calling you on the child inpatient rotation.

Identification of patient: I have a nine-year-old male named Doug Burton.

Reason patient presented: He was brought in by his mother after an incident in the home tonight, where he hit his three-year-old sister, drawing blood, and caused destruction of a lamp, table, and a window. He also had a school referral for hitting a peer. His mother said that she cannot guarantee safety in the home tonight.

Question to practitioner: Would you accept him for admission to inpatient?

Response from practitioner: Of course.

Vignette #9: A Previous Patient

Greeting: Dr. Thompson.

Self-identification: This is David at the Memorial Admission Department.

Purpose of call: I am calling you on a previous patient.

Identification of patient: Roger Jacobson has returned tonight requesting admission.

Reason patient presented: He had stopped taking his medication and reported command hallucinations telling him to kill himself and others.

Question to practitioner: Would you accept him for admission to inpatient?

Response from practitioner*:* Yes, of course.

Vignette #10: An Adult Referral to Intensive Outpatient/ Partial

Greeting: Dr. Bauer.

Self-identification: This is David at the Memorial Admission Department.

Purpose of call: I am calling you on the adult outpatient rotation.

Identification of patient: I interviewed Kay Henderson, a thirty-five-year-old female.

Reason patient presented: She reported having suicidal ideation with no plan earlier today, feeling hopeless, having poor sleep, and not able to do her housework.

Question to practitioner: Would you accept her for admission to partial?

Response from practitioner: Yes.

Vignette #11: An Adolescent Referral to Intensive Outpatient/Partial

Greeting: Dr. Bowman.

Self-identification: This is David at the Memorial Admission Department.

Purpose of call: I am calling you on the child-adolescent outpatient rotation.

Identification of patient: I interviewed Eileen Macy, a sixteen-year-old female.

Reason patient presented: She reported having suicidal ideation with no plan yesterday; feeling helpless, hopeless, and irritable; and having poor sleep.

Question to practitioner: Would you accept her for admission to the partial program?

Response from practitioner: Yes.

Vignette #12: A Follow-Up Call Requesting a Seventy-Two-Hour Hold

Greeting: Dr. Taylor.

Self-identification: This is David at the Memorial Admission Department.

Purpose of call: I am calling you back on Heidi Rife.

Identification of patient and problem: As discussed with you earlier, she reported that she had suicidal ideation with a plan earlier today and now she is requesting to leave.

Question to practitioner: Do you wish to put her on a seventy-two-hour hold?

Response from practitioner: Yes, put her on a hold.

Vignette #13: Requesting a Seventy-Two-Hour Hold Outright

Greeting: Dr. Taylor.

Self-identification: This is David at the Memorial Admission Department.

Purpose of call: I am calling you on the adult rotation.

Identification of patient and problem: I have a patient named Dan Krantz who was brought by a family member due to psychosis. The patient was uncooperative with the interview, responding to internal stimuli, and unable to answer any of the interview questions. The family member said that he went off of his medications and is using meth.

Question to practitioner: Will you admit him on a seventy-two-hour hold?

Response from practitioner: Yes, go ahead.

Vignette #14: A Complicated Child Case

Greeting: Dr. Thompson.

Self-identification: This is David at the Memorial Admission Department.

Purpose of call: I am calling you on something of a complicated case that will take me a bit longer to get through for the adolescent rotation.

Identification of patient and problem: John Boehner is a fourteen-year-old male brought in his mother and father after an incident in the home where he broke a glass light fixture, punched a hole in the wall, and then ran out of the house to be found about one hour later. His mother related that he said that he wanted to die but was not suicidal with plan. He also reported feeling hopeless and helpless, and he is having problems with sleep. His mother said that she has younger children in the home and said that she cannot keep things safe in the home.

Question to practitioner: Doctor, what is your leaning on this case? Is this inpatient or outpatient?

Response from practitioner: Admit to inpatient for safety.

Vignette #15: A Complicated Adult Case

Greeting: Dr. Taylor.

Self-identification: This is David at the Memorial Admission Department.

Purpose of call: I am calling you on something of a complicated case that will take me a bit longer to get through for the adult rotation.

Identification of patient and problem: Jennifer Deasy is a twenty-six-year-old female who presented tonight, reporting feeling hopeless and helpless. She reported that her boyfriend died yesterday from a heroin overdose, and she has not slept in two days because she herself has been using meth daily for the past few weeks (she could not be specific on the duration). She is reporting hearing voices and seeing hallucinations. She said that she was unsure if she was suicidal. She presented as paranoid and tangential but made it through the interview.

Question to practitioner: Doctor, what is your opinion on this case?

Response from practitioner: Admit to inpatient for safety.[8]

CONCLUDING THOUGHTS

This chapter discussed and modeled a script format in staffing cases with providers after the assessment interview. The script is a both a condensation and distillation of the interview data into the few necessary elements. The script specifies what criteria were present in the interview for or against admission to inpatient or an outpatient program. These scripts are applicable in most routine assessment cases.

The assessment clinician works in a tension of thoroughness versus brevity. The new clinician is challenged to condense all the information that took anywhere from fifteen minutes to hours to gather and phone a busy psychiatrist or provider who is likely multi-tasking or preoccupied. Initially, this process of experience or development can be emotionally overwhelming and mentally tiring, especially if the patient was difficult and the provider seems impatient over the phone. Given that a patient is in crisis, there is likely anxiety over missing some crucial information to the point of someone dying. Hopefully, the new clinician has some job orientation that includes shadowing an experienced clinician and observation of this process.

The average assessment clinician who perseveres is able to routinize and develop confidence in this practice with experience. Staffing with a provider is not necessarily a complicated process, but it is cognitively challenging, especially if there is limited job orientation.

The staffing process can be challenging for a mental health clinician in a rural area who is recruited to do occasional assessments at a local emergency department when the tendency is to refer a patient to a regional hospital that serves a catchment area.[9] This clinician may not get any job training from an experienced professional. The clinician may be staffing the case with an attending emergency physician who has limited training in mental health. Therefore, there can be an extra burden on the clinician who does not do this on a routine basis to be the consulting expert to be valid and accurate in reporting. Therefore, "thinking out" or routinely writing out a script in the manners suggested in this chapter can be helpful for the clinician especially when starting out in this work.

NOTES

1. Depending on the rules of the hospital, a provider may say that they only want a particular type of case the remainder of the night or say that they are not taking any more cases that day.
2. There are also sales scripts used by telemarketers.

3. Some practitioners do not accept certain types of patients. For example, some practitioners do not take addiction cases, patients who have limited English language skills, or cases on a court-ordered detention/commitment/mental inquest warrant. The assessment clinician would just go to the next provider on rotation.

4. The provider does not always take the lead in the effort of responding to the high utilizer's repeated seeking admission, and the provider may just be fatigued with such a patient. Furthermore, some hospitals adhere to the policy that a patient should be admitted if reporting being suicidal regardless of high utilization, and providers go along with it. It turns out that dealing with high utilizers is a case-by-case issue depending on insurance's continued willingness to pay, the aggression of the patient when admitted, and administration concerns.

5. The high utilizer who was just discharged may make the statement that they have not been on their medication in weeks. This easily proves to be a lie and an apparent attempt to manipulate when the clinician looks at the record and it shows the patient took medication yesterday or the same day. While the clinician will discover such a lie, it makes no sense to mention this to the patient or even confront the patient about the lie, as the clinician is not a moral authority.

6. Problematic high utilizers who are aggressive on units and in the admitting departments should be administratively addressed. There should be organizational protocols to prevent readmission for when the patient returns that have the support of risk managers and administrators. However, there is indeed the rare case where the clinician has confidence through repeated observation and experience that a certain anti-social high utilizer will not be an authentic danger to self despite the patient's verbal report; in the end, the clinician still is making a judgment call when going along with the recommendation not to admit.

7. An alternative script is "The patient reports suicidal ideation with no plan but she cannot contract for safety."

8. In the complicated cases, especially the "out of control" ones, some practitioners will direct assessment clinicians to seek prior authorization before accepting a patient. This has been common during fiscal strain, when a hospital has many "denied days" and trends of rigorous utilization management. This scenario is ethically questionable, and the clinician should seek direction from the supervisor or administrator on this practice. The standard should be patient safety versus whether prior authorization can be readily achieved. The facility, provider, and clinician could all be liable if the patient is not admitted merely because prior authorization is not granted by an insurance managed care organization.

9. With advances in internet coverage, software, and computer hardware, there has been a trend of using telehealth assessments in rural hospitals, lessening the burden on local resources. Large healthcare systems with multiple hospitals are using telehealth where an experienced assessment clinician in a central location can conduct the interview for outposts. Rural hospitals or healthcare systems have started to contract with mental health hospitals in metropolitan areas to do assessment interviews by telehealth. Nevertheless, there can be budgetary and clinical situations that require a local, face-to-face interview. A psychotic individual is difficult to interview over telehealth and usually necessitates a qualified clinician in situ.

Chapter 11

Telling People "No"

A reality of the hospital and emergency assessment is that not everyone meets the criteria for admission to inpatient or any other level of care. The significance of this reality varies according to the situation, patient agenda, and the array of services that a hospital organization offers to the community.

Officials, authorities, agencies, and other organizations refer individuals for assessment for matters that are not crises and that do not necessitate inpatient admission. Legal and correctional authorities will order those on probation and parole to get screened for mental health, substance use, and possible treatment. School officials prompt parents to have children assessed after behavioral incidents. Child protective services will refer both parents and children for screening and treatment of identified problems and issues. Rehabs and halfway houses send adults who have been actively using to get screened for detox as a prerequisite for admission to those programs. The psychiatric hospital admission department can be viewed and utilized locally as an additional assessment arm of other agencies.

The outcome of many of these mandated assessments is that the patient does not meet criteria for inpatient but maybe lower levels of care. The patient and families frequently expect these outcomes as they are merely coming as an act of compliance. They will take the assessment documentation and leave without incident.

However, there is the patient, or other family member (usually parent-figure), who reveals an agenda of admission when criteria are not met. Because of the agenda, the interaction changes in character from a task-oriented, fact-finding interview to an emotional exchange where the patient or family member will use intimidation tactics that can include:

- blaming the clinician for the problem.
- personally attacking the clinician with insults and name-calling.
- stalling the clinician with a series of Why? Why? Why? questions.
- making self-pity statements that imply the clinician is being cruel or sadistic.
- quibbling or debating with the clinician about the legitimacy of the assessment.
- making veiled or explicit threats (It will be on you!).

Often, the clinician must go in circles to explain the reason for the recommendation of a lower level of care and tolerate the patient's emotional pleas and tactics.

The emotional encounter can go further as the patient or family member not getting admitted may instigate a triangle of drama (see figure 11.1).[1] The drama starts when they complain to others in the waiting room or another clinician or demand to see the supervisor. The nature of the complaint can escalate and evolve into a personal attack on the clinician in front of an audience.

Depending on the composition[2] of the audience in the hallway or waiting room, the angry patient or family member can stir up a crowd that joins in the anger. This has the potential to be a battle of potential humiliation and intimidation of the clinician in front of other patients, families, and peers. The clinician is challenged in these cases to maintain professional composure.

Composure in these challenging situations is demonstrated by the practices of assertiveness and boundaries. Assertiveness and boundary setting are professional skills that can be developed and are the focus of this chapter. This chapter will discuss personal boundaries and their integration with assertiveness and then demonstrate their application through practice vignettes.

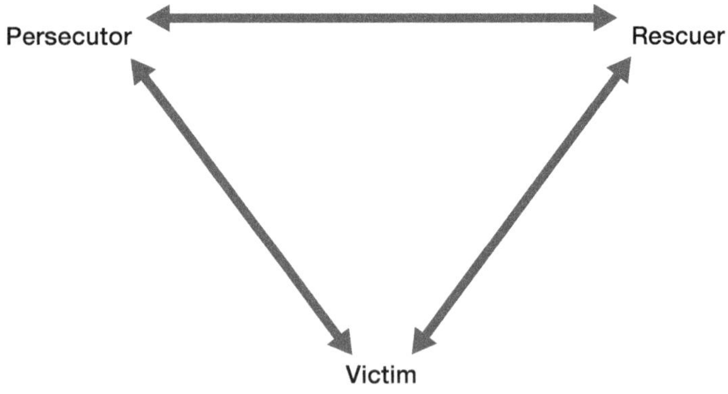

Figure 11.1. SB Karpman's Drama Triangle.

REVIEWING BOUNDARIES

As discussed in chapter 3, boundaries are lines or limits between individuals. They can be expressed relationally in multiple ways. Figure 11.2 depicts these boundaries. The closer the more personal and emotional the relationship, the fewer boundaries exist.

How these boundaries are maintained is key to the order and stability in the relationships between two or more people. Violation of these boundaries tends to elicit a variation of anxiety or anger resulting in chaos.[3] However, emotion felt in reaction to violations tends to guide one or more people in an automatic fashion to adjust and re-establish boundaries.[4]

There are interpersonal boundaries and then there are professional boundaries as discussed earlier. As discussed in chapter 3, the assessment interview logically crosses interpersonal boundaries but has the feature of intentional confidentiality to compensate. Furthermore, the licensed professional-patient relationship in general has legally defined boundaries to protect the patient. While assessment clinicians are not required to be credentialed professionals in all jurisdictions, it is imperative that the clinician seek to practice boundaries with patients and family members, especially when telling a patient that they are not being admitted to inpatient.

For all intents and purposes, the salient boundaries (as depicted in figure 11.2) when a patient or family member is escalating are *actions*, *information*, *time*, and *emotions*. While it seems unlikely that they have insight in what they are doing, they are essentially:

1. attempting to intimidate the clinician to act in their favor despite the lack of criteria.
2. seeking an explanation that renders more information than appropriate.

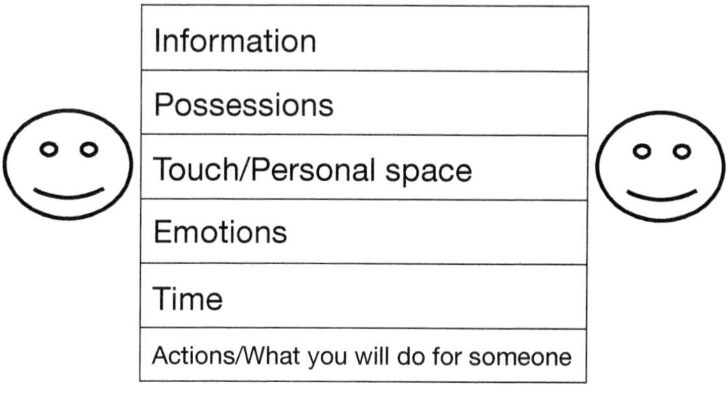

Figure 11.2. Basic Boundaries.

3. occupying more of the clinician's time.
4. drawing the clinician into an emotional encounter that can lead to loss of composure and a continuation of #1, #2, and #3.

This is a situation where there is a distinction between reacting and responding. Reacting is an impulsive, emotional utterance or expression. Responding is a rational, measured answer to the situation or other person. Reacting can lead to an emotional tug of war between the parties in the encounter which tends to escalate further in emotional intensity and volume to the potential of physical altercation. Responding is, instead, emotionally contradicting the escalated patient or parent. Depending on their psychopathology and degree of intoxication the escalated individuals can likely de-escalate.

Again, returning to the concepts discussed in chapter 3, transactional analysis has much to illuminate in these emotional situations and how the clinician can maintain professional boundaries. Transactional analysis recognizes three ego or emotional states that exist in relational transactions: parent, child, and adult. The individual who has escalated to the point of yelling is demonstrating or exhibiting a child ego state. The parent ego state is complementary to the child ego state as it can equally be an emotional reaction when giving (or perceived as giving) direction, criticism, or chastisement (see figure 11.3). Regardless of clinician intent, the more pathological or intoxicated the escalated patient or parent is, the higher the likelihood will be that any response

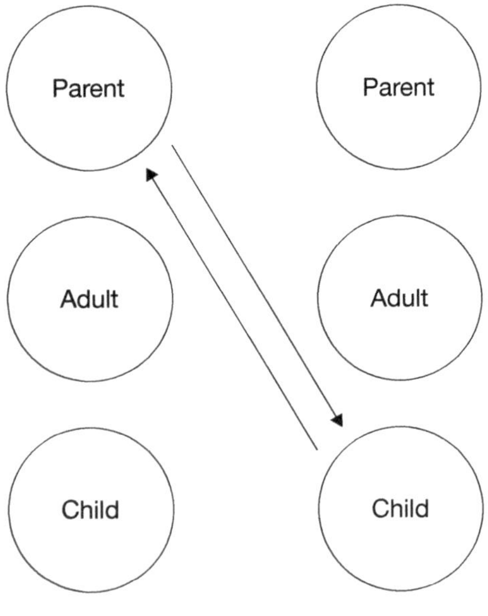

Figure 11.3. Parent-Child Dyad in TA.

will be perceived as patronizing and demeaning in nature with a potential of further escalation.

Nevertheless, the clinician's best emotional response in these situations is to exhibit or demonstrate an adult ego or emotional state by a tone, volume, and facial expression of "modified boredom" as an outward demonstration of calmness. Modified boredom and calmness are not the same internal, emotional states, but outwardly, they look and sound the same and can position the clinician in a place of emotional power in the encounter with an escalated individual. Modified boredom also can come across as confidence, rational detachment, and courage.

Modified boredom is truly a pragmatic script as it is a planned and practiced response for the new clinician. It is a starting point that with experience evolves into confident calmness. The elements of modified boredom include

1. a conversational volume of voice that may be almost a whisper depending on the character pathology of the patient,
2. a lack of emotion in tone,
3. a plain facial affect/expression,
4. a relaxed but not slumping stance,[5] and
5. a socially distanced space of at least six feet when possible.

Modified boredom also includes use of fewer words. With the use of fewer words, the clinician is forced to listen and think more, and be measured in word choice. Word choice can be adapted from the style of assertive communication.

UNDERSTANDING ASSERTIVENESS

Assertiveness is a combination of belief system, behavior, and communication style with the intent of respectfully standing up for your rights without denying the other person/people their rights. It is considered a healthy manner of communicating. In contrast, the unhealthy communication styles are the following:

- Aggressive: Standing up for rights and wants in a way that is at the expense of others
- Passive: Indirectly standing up or not at all standing up for one's rights
- Passive-aggressive: Not standing up for your rights, and then out of acting in an aggressive fashion in another way

Professional communication in the context of the assessment is direct, assertive communication that respects the patient's right to appropriate treatment and the necessary information.

Assertiveness starts with beliefs. It is either impeded by traditional but mistaken beliefs or driven by assertive rights. Table 11.1 shows a contrast of these types of beliefs. The traditional beliefs are a variation of the cognitive distortions labeled "shoulds-musts-oughts." Such cognitive distortions are emotional and not rational thinking. Given how stressful an emotional encounter might be, there is the natural tendency to indeed think with mistaken but traditional beliefs and give into the patient's manipulative pleas despite the lack of objective criteria for admission. Assertive rights are in sum a mindful, philosophical foundation that supports the setting and maintenance of professional-patient boundaries.

Assertive behavior is demonstrated by "I" statements or scripts. These are planned and rehearsed statements. Basic I statements begin with some formulation of I think, I feel, or I want. They can be more complex clinician responses such as the following:

- I have done a complete assessment, and our recommendation for you is . . .
- I can see that you do not agree. Is there something else you wish to add?
- I respect your right to your feelings on this, but you did not meet criteria.
- I observe that you are angry, and you can be angry, but this is the treatment recommendation.

Table 11.1. Mistaken versus Assertive Belief

Mistaken, Traditional Beliefs	*Assertive Rights*
You must always try to accommodate others. If you don't, they won't be there when you need them.	You have a right to say "no."
You must always have a good reason for what you feel and do.	You have a right not to have to justify yourself to others.
When someone is in trouble, you must help them.	You have a right not to take responsibility for someone else's problem.
You must be sensitive to the needs and wishes of others, even when they are unable to tell you what they want.	You have the right not to have to anticipate others' needs and wishes.
It's always a good policy to stay on people's good side.	You have a right not to have to worry about the goodwill of others.
It's not nice to put people off. If questioned, give an answer.	You have a right to choose not to respond to a situation.

- I want to recommend the treatment that you qualify for today, and it just happens to be the intensive outpatient program (IOP).
- I have listened to you, and I need to move on so we will show you out.

Assertiveness avoids starting sentences with "you" as it comes across as aggressive.

When dealing with escalated patients or family members (especially parental figures) who are demonstrating intense anger because they or their children are not being admitted, the emotional interaction can be an argument that evidences to be gamey and manipulative on their part. The patient often may just end the need for further interaction by adding that they are suicidal and will kill themselves by a certain method if not admitted and will "win" inpatient admission. Also, the parent may create or add additional information that makes the child meet criteria. However, not all will add additional claims and will instead just continue to argue by personally attacking the clinician in some manner.

When it comes to parental figures who are escalated over their child not being admitted, they may continue to seek to "win." This includes asking to see a manager or supervisor, but they may persist in arguing with the clinician, which includes making personal attacks.

Options for assertive responses the clinician can use with the arguing patient or parent include the following:

- *Sound like a broken record.* (When someone will not take "no" for an answer.) Choose a simple/concise sentence and repeat it repeatedly like a broken record. *Example: Your child did not meet criteria for admission today.*
- *Make a content-to process shift.* Shift the discussion from the topic to an analysis of what is going on between the two of you. *Example: We are getting off the point.*
- *Assertive agreement.* Acknowledge criticism with which you agree. Here you do not need to explain unless you wish to. *Example: You are right. You did report that.*
- *Clouding.* When someone is putting you down as a person, acknowledge something in the criticism with which you can agree, agree in part, or agree in principle, and ignore the rest. You rephrase the critical person's words so that you can honestly concur (not agree but concur). By giving the appearance of agreeing without promising to change, the critic runs out of reasons to criticize you. Example: (agree in part) *You are right. You said that you were detoxing.* (Agree in the probability) *You may be right that I missed something.* (Agree in the principle) *If we missed things as often as you say, it certainly would be a problem.*

- *Painting the issue.* When someone becomes defensive and personalizes when you make an assertive request in negotiating for something. Example: *This is not an issue of whether I don't care that you have a heroin addiction. This is an issue of admission criteria being met.*

One other internal strategy in telling an arguing patient or parent "no" is for the clinician to "slow down" and focus on listening instead of trying to get a point across. This strategy assumes that a gamey patient or parent is not necessarily listening and the clinician will not prove a point, so it is best to maintain an emotional boundary. If the clinician can slow down and demonstrate use of modified boredom and assertive statements, the emotional boundary becomes evident between the clinician and the escalating individual.

While it may seem optimal for the clinician to manage the interaction with the escalating patient or parent, there is nothing wrong with a clinician handing them over to a supervisor or lead. The supervisor or lead is not a direct object of anger (like the clinician may have become) and may have a stronger position in de-escalation and getting the patient and family exited from the admitting department. Prior to the supervisor taking over, it is crucial that the clinician apprises the supervisor *how* the admission criteria was not met, so a consistent clinical stance can be maintained.

Despite the modified boredom and the assertiveness, there can be a point in the process where any further attempt to explain is fruitless and only adding proverbial fuel to the fire. When the escalated individual is neither providing any new clinical information nor accepting the polite and assertive statement of limit, the clinician or supervisor may need to use the process to content shift technique to refocus the discussion or set the next limit and walk away with or without warning.

Frequently, escalated patients or parents ironically make claims to the in situ audience (the others there at the moment) that the clinician or supervisor was being rude for doing so, but it is usually obvious that the former was neither polite nor civil to the latter.[6] The exact timing of leaving the conversation is a matter of personal judgment, but what matters is that the professional is mindful, rational, and responding versus merely emotionally reacting.

VIGNETTES

The following are vignettes depicting situations where the clinician has to say no and inform the patient or family member of a recommendation other than admission to inpatient. A review of the assertive techniques used will be discussed at the end of each vignette.

Vignette #1: The Person Not Meeting Criteria for Detox

A forty-five-year-old male presented seeking inpatient treatment to detox from alcohol. This individual reported being depressed, and he had been consuming eight beers daily to self-medicate. His last use was of four twelve-ounce beers just prior to coming in to the intake center. He blew a blood alcohol level of 0.125. He denied a prior history of complicated withdrawal (e.g., withdrawal seizures, delirium tremens) and any current withdrawal symptoms. Regarding the mental health screening questions, he denied suicidal ideation, homicidal ideation, and psychosis.

The clinician staffed the case with the next physician on rotation, and the conclusion was the patient did not meet criteria for inpatient detox. The recommendation was for the patient to be referred to the hospital's IOP. The clinician met with the patient back in the interview room to discuss the recommendation and give the referral paperwork for IOP.

Clinician: Thank you, sir, for your patience while I staffed your case with one of our hospital physicians. After reviewing your assessment against our facility criteria, you do not qualify for hospital admission at this time.

Patient: This is bulls--t. I guess you guys just don't like helping people, do you?

Clinician: Of course we do. We are required to follow rules, however, in terms of what we can recommend. We cannot simply admit everyone. A referral to our IOP is all we can offer at this time; however, this is a great program with a high success rate.

Patient: Okay, well what are the rules? Why the f--k don't I "qualify"?

Clinician: Unfortunately, we are not allowed to release our admission criteria; however, in your case it turns out your level of active withdrawal was not significant enough to warrant admission.

Patient: But don't you think that's bulls--t? You got people out here looking for help and you're denying them that opportunity.

Clinician: Sir, we are not denying you the opportunity to receive treatment. We have offered you a referral to our IOP. And our criteria are set against treatment programs that will best serve your needs currently.

The patient evidenced continued irritability and made a gesture of exasperation but signed the referral form for the IOP.[7] The patient then left the facility without any further outburst or incident.

In this vignette, the clinician painted the issue and clarified the standard being used. The patient evidenced anger and was argumentative, but by using modified boredom and maintaining a boundary of information, the clinician was able to keep the interaction short and time-limited.

Vignette #2: The Malingerer Who Will Not Say Enough

A thirty-one-year-old female with a history of numerous admissions for suicidal ideation presented again to the psychiatric hospital reporting she had been feeling down as of late due to several stressors including a divorce from a few years ago, housing issues, and an ongoing custody battle. The patient's affect was mostly flat interspersed with periods of upbeat mood. The woman "sadly" reported today that she did not want to live any longer but denied a plan or intent of suicide.

The clinician inquired further whether the woman had started to do anything suggesting suicidal thoughts including giving away belongings, writing a will, or having collected pills. The patient denied having done those things. After the interview, the clinician staffed the case with the previous psychiatrist who recommended outpatient treatment. The clinician informed the patient of the recommendation and the following ensued.

Patient: What? No. I need that inpatient treatment. I told you; I don't want to live any longer.

Clinician: Yes ma'am. I wrote that down but during our extended conversation you told me you had no plan or intent on harming or killing yourself. On that, you unfortunately do not qualify for admission.

Patient: Where am I supposed to stay tonight? I'm homeless right now and that's part of the reason I am depressed. I wanted to come here to get straightened out for a few days.

Clinician: I can refer you to a shelter for tonight and once you start your outpatient treatment with us, your case manager can assist you with finding a solution to your housing dilemma.

Patient: I still don't know why I am not being admitted. Is it because I've been here so many times or what?

Clinician: No. We don't base our treatment recommendations on how many times you have been here. You're not being recommended for inpatient admission because your responses to the assessment questions do not warrant the need for admission stabilization.

The incongruity between the patient's report of depressive symptoms and her actual presentation of positive emotion caused the clinician to be skeptical if this patient may be malingering. Many malingerers become savvy by experience to say that they are suicidal with a plan that they have access to, such as running out into the street, and so they succeed in getting admitted. The patient could have changed her answer and said that she did have a plan to get admitted and have a place to stay. In this case, she played either the ignorant victim or stupid card ("I still don't know why I am not being admitted") and the clinician used a form of the broken record to avoid queuing the patient into upping the ante.

Vignette #3: The Eating Disordered Adolescent

A fourteen-year-old girl was brought in by her parents for assessment on a Friday night. The girl had a history of bulimia and was in an afterschool program for eating disorders. She had a history of purging or inducing vomiting after eating candy (sugar was a trigger) and on the day of assessment she was given a small packet of candy by someone and she had eaten it.

In this case, it served to note that the patient was medically stable within the screening practices of the admitting department. She had a normal blood pressure and pulse. She denied being in any pain and did not appear to be in any physical distress.

The narrative of the events reported by both the patient and the mother proved to be a power struggle. The patient showed the candy wrapper to her parents after she had consumed the candy. Her mother then said that she and the girl's father told her that they had to watch her to make sure she did not purge. The patient then ran from the house, but then denied purging today. The mother said she called the patient's outpatient therapist who recommended that the daughter be made safe and under observation for the weekend given the consumption of candy and the likelihood of bulimic purging.

The girl herself denied suicidal ideation, homicidal ideation, and psychosis. She reported feeling hopeless and helpless. The case was staffed with the next provider on rotation who recommended that the patient be referred to the child-adolescent IOP.

Clinician: *(Addressing the parents)* I have staffed your case with the next psychiatrist on the rotation and our recommendation is for her to be referred to the IOP.

Mother: Why? She has put herself in the hospital with chemical imbalance before due to her purging. She needs to be in the hospital tonight.

Clinician: Tonight, she is not meeting criteria.

Mother: I am not going to sit all weekend watching her. You must admit her!

Clinician: She is not meeting criteria.

Mother: You have no idea of what I go through with this eating disorder s--t. I want to talk to the doctor!

Clinician: Ma'am, I am confident that the doctor is not going to talk with you or any parent in this situation. Because they tell us they won't.

Mother: You've screwed up. If you did your job right, she would be admitted.

Clinician: You may be right that I missed something. In a nutshell, someone gave her a fun size package of candy. She ate it. She showed you that she ate it. You told her that you had to watch her because of her history of purging. She ran from the house. She came back after fifteen minutes. You brought her in for assessment given her history of bulimic behaviors. She denied suicidal ideation, and you have not heard her make any such comments. She denied wanting to kill anyone. She denied hearing any voices or seeing anything. She reported feeling hopeless and helpless. Her sleep is good. Her appetite is fair. Was there something else?

Mother: She needs to be admitted!

Clinician: I told the doctor your statement and your concern about her needing to be watched the whole weekend to prevent purging, and he directed referral to the outpatient program. Here is the form, if you would please sign it, and I'll show you out.

Mother: I'm not signing anything! I WANT TO TALK WITH YOUR SUPERVISOR!

The clinician apprised the supervisor of the situation and the clinical content, and the case was turned over to the supervisor. The clinician heard the mother say, "It's on you if something happens to my daughter." After about twenty minutes of talking with the supervisor, the girl and her parents left the facility.

This case appeared to be a family dynamic issue where the girl and her parents, especially her mother, were engaged in both a power struggle and attention-seeking and pushed successfully her parents' "buttons." The mother demonstrated an agenda of not wanting to be inconvenienced by the requirement of spending her weekend directly observing her daughter for bulimic purging and demonstrated an entitled demeanor in attempting to intimidate the clinician.

The clinician used broken record and clouding ("may be") to respond to the mother's child-level personal attack. As part of the clouding technique, the clinician stayed on the adult level of emotion and briefly reviewed with the mother, father, and patient the crucial points that also would eventually be the written summary of the assessment.

It does not mean that the clinician failed in setting boundaries and being assertive when the mother demanded to talk with the supervisor. The mother was not being reasonable; she was emotionally escalated and likely evidenced symptoms of a personality disorder herself, and the clinician was neither going to satisfy nor convince her.

Does it mean that the mother did not have a valid concern? Her daughter's eating disorder was a valid concern, but the mother demonstrated having her own emotional issues that appeared to impair her own abilities to cope with and manage this situation by observing her daughter for the whole weekend. Bringing her daughter to get the hospital to observe her daughter was a way to escape this responsibility that she lacked in emotional ability to fulfill and so she tried to manipulate the clinician and the hospital to handle it.

Vignette #4: The Parental Figure Trying to Use the Hospital as Punishment and Respite

A grandmother brought her eight-year-old grandson in for assessment. He had been having increasing problems at school, including getting into a fight earlier in the day. He also had knocked over a lamp at home just prior to coming to the hospital. The grandmother said that she could not handle the grandson and that he needed to be hospitalized.

During the interview, the clinician had established that the boy had been with the grandmother for about two months. The grandmother got custody due to her daughter/patient's mother being arrested and the patient being placed in foster care for several months. The patient had never hit anyone in the home nor had he committed any prior property damage; the patient had been engaging in horseplay with a cousin also living in the home. The patient had previously been on stimulant medication for attention deficit hyperactivity disorder, and the grandmother stated that she decided that the patient did not need to be taking it, especially because it required her to go to the pediatrician monthly to get the prescription.

The patient did not evidence meeting criteria for inpatient admission. He denied suicidal ideation, homicidal ideation, and psychosis. He seemed to be restless and inattentive in the grandmother's presence. When the clinician met with him alone to answer the abuse questions, the patient seemed to be pleasant and cooperative. The clinician reviewed the case with a psychiatrist on the phone and the treatment recommendation was for the patient to go to the hospital's outpatient program or for the grandmother to take the patient back to the pediatrician for attention deficit hyperactivity disorder medication.

> **Clinician:** I've staffed the case with the next psychiatrist, Dr. Miller, and we have a recommendation of your grandson either coming to our partial hospitalization program or you taking him back to the pediatrician to get his attention deficit hyperactivity disorder medication.

Grandmother: That's not going to work. I can't handle him. He's a danger to other people in the household.

Clinician: So, let's step back and review. I may have missed something. What is he doing that is a danger in the household?

Grandmother: He's breaking things!

Clinician: In the interview, you said that he had broken a lamp. What else did he break?

Grandmother: Oh, I don't know! I just can't handle him!

Clinician: Ma'am, with everything you and he had reported, he does not meet criteria to be in the hospital.

Grandmother: He needs to be in the hospital!

Clinician: He does not meet the criteria to be in.

Grandmother: If something worse happens, it's on you! I want to talk to your supervisor.

The clinician briefed the supervisor and turned the matter over to the supervisor. The supervisor talked with the grandmother. The clinician could hear the grandmother screaming and criticizing the clinician. The grandmother left a few minutes later with the patient, having refused to sign the treatment recommendation forms.

This appeared to be a case where a personality-disordered grandparent was being saddled with the care of grandchildren. One of those grandchildren, the patient who has attention deficit hyperactivity disorder, was benefiting from the medication, but it either inconvenienced her or she was too overwhelmed to attend all the details of the care of her grandchildren. Nevertheless, the patient was having behavioral problems related to not having his medication.

The patient may have met criteria for admission if he had been physically aggressive toward others in the house to include injury or had threatened a family member with some kind of weapon-like object. However, none of that kind of information was disclosed. While in discussion with the grandmother, the clinician gave her one more chance to report (or maybe even fabricate) additional information, but she did not, and so the treatment recommendation continued to be appropriate.

The assertiveness techniques that the clinician used included "broken record" and shift from content to process. The clinician repeated the fact that the patient did not meet criteria for inpatient but reopened the assessment process for gathering additional information.

Vignette #5: An Angry Patient Instigating Drama by Drawing in a Third Person

A twenty-eight-year-old female with multiple previous admissions came in alone for an assessment for detox. The patient was just discharged five days before this assessment. The patient reported that she had resumed consumption of alcohol three days ago and that she had been consuming one pint per day and she blew a blood alcohol level of 0.109. She denied being suicidal or homicidal, or having psychosis. She reported being hopeless and helpless. She denied any current detox symptoms and had no prior history of complicated withdrawal.

The clinician staffed the case with the previous psychiatrist and the recommendation was for the patient to go to the IOP. The clinician organized the referral papers and went to tell the patient. The patient was in the hallway.

Clinician: I talked with Dr. Michaels, and our recommendation is for you to go to the IOP.

Patient: No! I relapsed and I started drinking again. I am going to go through detox. If I don't come into the hospital, I am going to die from withdrawal!

Clinician: Yes, I hear you, but you have just gotten discharged and the doctor said that you have not been using for long enough to be going through detox. At this time, your symptoms are meeting criteria for the IOP. Do you have a way to go home? Or do you need me to arrange for a cab?

Patient: I need to be admitted!

Clinician: I am sorry, but you are just not meeting criteria. Shall I arrange for a cab?

Patient: I'll take the cab.

Clinician: Do you want to go to the address that you put on the face sheet?

Patient: *(sighing)* Yes.

The clinician went and got the cab voucher and called for a ride. The clinician went back out to the waiting room. The patient and another female (also a high utilizer well-known to the staff) present for assessment came up together and confronted the clinician.

Other female: *(Loudly)* You're not going to admit her? She's going to get sick and die!

Clinician: I am not allowed to discuss another patient with you.

Other female: *(Screaming)* YOU DON'T CARE ABOUT HER!

Clinician: I am glad that you care, but, again, I can't discuss another patient with you.

Clinician: *(to patient)* I've called your cab. I'll show you out.

The clinician showed the patient out and returned to the office to finish paperwork. The other female came to the office door, knocked, and demanded to talk to the clinician.

Other female: YOU ARE GOING TO BE RESPONSIBLE FOR HER DYING!

Clinician: I hear your concern, but again, I am not allowed to discuss another patient's business, especially if there is no release of information.

Other female: YOU ARE A TERRIBLE PERSON!

Clinician: I am sorry you feel that way. Is there anything else I can do for you? Some water or something? Otherwise, I have to get back to work.

Other female: I CAN'T STAND YOU!

In this case, the clinician was aware that the third person (other female) involved was part of the in situ audience and was not related to the patient being assessed and was able to set boundaries immediately and minimize the drama by being a broken record in a modified boredom manner. If the clinician was not familiar with who the third person was, the clinician should have asked. Otherwise, the drama happened instantaneously because the third person was a personality-disordered individual with anger management issues and poor emotional boundaries. The anger management problem and poor emotional boundaries contributed to impulsive codependency of either a total stranger or relative stranger's problem in a loud, disruptive demeanor that became another issue for the clinician to respond to and manage.

Vignette #6: After the Fact Family Member Phone Call

A forty-three-year-old female presented for assessment. She said that she had been dropped off at the hospital by her mother. There was no collateral information given on this individual prior to her being seen.

In the interview, the patient said that she had been suicidal five days ago in which she took an overdose of pills but still woke up. The patient said that she had thoughts of wanting to go to sleep and not wake up four days ago, but she denied any suicidal ideation in the past seventy-two hours. Furthermore, she denied homicidal ideation and psychosis but she felt somewhat hopeless and helpless with poor sleep and appetite. The patient said that she would do what the hospital recommended.

The clinician called the next provider on rotation, and the treatment recommendation was that the patient be referred to the partial hospitalization program. The patient signed the referral form and left the facility.

After the patient left, the patient's mother called and demanded to talk to the clinician by name.

Clinician: Hello.

Mother: You just saw my daughter, Valerie Wayne. You should have admitted her. She's suicidal!

Clinician: Ma'am, I can neither confirm nor deny the identity of anyone here without a release of information. Furthermore, I cannot confirm that you are who you say you are.

Mother: She took a bunch of pills last night to kill herself.

Clinician: Ma'am, if that is the case it looks like you will need to take her to the emergency room for medical treatment and consider filing a petition for involuntary admission.

Mother: She was in your assessment room, and you let her out!

Clinician: Ma'am, again I cannot confirm or deny the presence of any patient.

Mother: I brought her in because she needed help, but I left.

Clinician: Ma'am, if that was indeed the case, you should have stayed or made a phone call in advance so we would have had the information. But again, if you have that situation, I recommend that you take her to an emergency room or go file a court petition to have her picked up and assessed.

This is a common and unsolvable drama where a family member calls after the interview with additional clinical information that is essentially useless since the assessed patient is gone from the hospital. The family member is essentially calling up playing a rescuer telling the clinician that they did wrong by not admitting the patient.

The clinician is limited because there was no release of information to talk with the complaining family member. In this situation the clinician can only be a broken record and assertively suggest in generalities what options exist for the family member to address the issue.

CONCLUDING THOUGHTS

The matter of telling people that they or their family member does not meet the criteria to get admitted is a regular part of the job. When the assessment is sought due to an official mandate such as from the school, court, or child welfare worker, the answer of "no" may be a welcome disposition. However, it becomes a professional and emotional challenge when either the patient or parental figure has an agenda of the patient getting admitted and criteria is not met.

Emotional intelligence, especially in the realm of assessment, is both a skill set and capacity that is not necessarily appreciated by all who seek to work in the helping professions. However, it is at the heart of demonstrated professionalism by which one succeeds, sustains, and reduces the likelihood of avoiding burnout. A clinician's emotional intelligence (or the lack thereof) is demonstrated in the face of the drama and conflict that comes when telling an angry and manipulative patient or parental figure that they are not being admitted.

Emotional intelligence involves appreciating the dimensions and dynamics of the unpleasant interaction. The angry adult's behavior can be interpreted as a child within Berne's framework of transactional analysis. The clinician should technically play the game in responding in a modified bored tone of voice that comes across as an adult. The tone of voice has great emotional power in the exchange in both setting a boundary and assisting in defusing the situation.

Furthermore, the clinician can set boundaries or limits by using the rehearsed scripts of assertiveness in the tone of modified boredom. Modified boredom is itself a boundary in this case because the clinician is not contributing to the emotional escalation but will either contribute to de-escalation or elucidate the patient's pathology, toxicity, and emotional immaturity that may just need to be redirected or plainly ignored.

Nevertheless, there is still the possibility of the exchange escalating into the emotional conflict of drama. This is where the patient or parent acts as a victim and triangulates one or more other "rescuers" into the interaction because they did not get inpatient admission for themselves or their child. While it is hard not to take it personally and react in a similar emotional fashion, the professional clinician should be rehearsed for such situations to demonstrate assertiveness and boundaries that present as a rational, professional response.

NOTES

1. S. B. Karpman, 2014, *A game free life. The definitive book on the drama triangle and compassion triangle by the originator and author. The new transactional analysis of intimacy, openness, and happiness*, San Francisco: Drama Triangle Publications.

2. Other individuals in the waiting room with poor emotional boundaries and general irritability from their own intoxication, detox discomfort, and mental health

issues can feed into the drama and make statements of complaint that appear to "rescue" the victim.

3. For example, someone sharing too much information of a sexual nature (often called too much information or TMI) can elicit the anxiety of embarrassment or the anger of disgust. Getting hugged without permission (a violation of the space boundary) usually elicits irritation or anger.

4. For example, someone making a strange or angry statement elicits reactions of discomfort or bemusement that lead to the hearer stopping and pausing or slightly backing away.

5. Some agencies and organizations may subscribe to a safety/crisis intervention system that has a prescribed script for verbal and emotional escalation that includes a definition and description for what an appropriate posture and stance looks like. If the clinician works in such an organization using a particular system, compliance with that system is encouraged.

6. An in situ audience only develops if there is emotional contagion. Emotional contagion happens when there are others with poor emotional boundaries and high emotional reactivity.

7. Alcohol can intensify emotional states and reactions.

Chapter 12

Insurance Prior Authorizations

It can be taxing enough to interview a difficult patient and then mentally switch gears to staff the case with a less than pleasant provider, but the clinician then usually has yet another challenge after that: to get a prior authorization. While not applicable in all situations, an assessment clinician in the United States is usually required to seek "prior authorization" or "pre-certification" from the insurance carrier or managed care organization (MCO).[1,2] Prior authorization is the act of approval by a payor source that an admission meets criteria for the medical service being rendered. In this case, the clinician is pressed to demonstrate to the MCO, insurance company, or government agency[3] that the patient meets criteria for admission and the hospital should be reimbursed for services rendered.

There are three formats for seeking prior authorization: phone call, fax, and online form. MCOs and insurance companies can change their format for prior authorizations over time or even go back and forth on their preferences.[4] There can be significant changes in those formats from long forms to short forms based on key indicators.[5] Each manner of prior authorization has its easy points and pitfalls based on the strength of the clinician.

In a grand sense with prior authorization, the roles are reversed; the assessment clinician is being interviewed, tested, and scrutinized as to

1. the quality of their interviewing skills,
2. the quality of clinical judgment demonstrated,
3. whether the insurance company/MCO or other payor source agrees with the treatment recommendation,
4. their writing skills and how well they fill out a form, and
5. whether the payor source will approve the admission for potential payment.[6]

There can be dread when a particular insurance shows up on a patient's forms because of the rigor or difficulty involved. The insurance carriers or subcontracting MCOs have different patterns of utilization management or review which means more questions and/or difficult questions.

Also, the prior authorization process is very human. The different MCO reviewers bring their personalities to the interaction which could include editorializing, arguing, and what feels like personal criticism of the clinician. The conversation with the reviewer can come across as a negotiation as to why the insurance should grant prior authorization.

This chapter will discuss prior authorizations. It will start with a definition and review the context of prior authorizations within utilization management. It will then discuss skills and strategies for gaining successful prior authorizations.

PRIOR AUTHORIZATION AS AN ELEMENT OF UTILIZATION MANAGEMENT

Utilization management is a set of insurance cost-control practices. Essentially insurers began to scrutinize healthcare providers for justification for medical services and whether billed services were being delivered. Quality was also part of the scrutiny as insurers were only going to pay for necessary services that were approved. Utilization management standards are generally shaped by research data which may also be called "evidence-based" or "best" practice.[7]

For the purpose of clarity, there is often an interchanging of the terms *utilization review* and *utilization management*. It is fair to say that to the average allied healthcare professional, both forms refer to the same burden of proving treatment criteria is met or was met to get reimbursement. However, there is a distinction between the two terms in that *utilization management* is conducted in real time while the patient is present and *utilization review* is after the patient has been discharged or after the medical services have been rendered.

In the US context,[8] utilization review is a cost-control practice that was initially used by the federal government in the 1960s to control Medicare and Medicaid costs.[9] It became a dominant practice in the commercial insurance industry to maximize profits and improve quality.[10] States have intermittently used utilization management and review for Medicaid funds as part of fiscal control practices often referred to as "capitation."[11] Utilization management and review became dominant with the passage of the Affordable Care Act in 2010 when more people became eligible for Medicaid; states are still limited in what they can contribute to the program, and it was all the more essential to manage those funds.[12]

Prior authorization is the opening phase of utilization management. It is where the insurer or MCO issues a determination as to whether it will grant initial approval of an admission to the level of care that is being sought. In most "live" prior authorization encounters, the clinician will hear a disclaimer from the reviewer that payment is not guaranteed based on the rest of utilization review process.

Assuming a prior authorization is granted, the MCO will then conduct "concurrent" reviews to determine whether a patient continues to meet criteria to be in the hospital. It becomes incumbent upon the hospital to demonstrate to the MCO that the patient both needs continued treatment and is benefitting from it.[13] If such proof is not provided, the MCO may issue a denial for any further certification of days in the hospital.[14]

An MCO also may conduct retrospective review after a patient is discharged to determine whether standards of care were met and payment for services is disbursed to the provider. So assessment clinicians are not solely responsible for whether the hospital gets paid, but it is incumbent that they successfully execute the prior authorization.

The prior authorization process can challenge the clinician's mental stamina, especially after difficult assessments. The clinician may have to be on the phone with an MCO reviewer up to one hour, where the clinician's work can be scrutinized. Some MCO reviewers can be argumentative and judgmental to the point of being rude. The clinician can walk away feeling exhausted and burned out from the whole process of one case while it may be early in the shift with more assessments to conduct.

THE PHONE CALL PRIOR AUTHORIZATION

The phone call tends to be the most dreaded version of the prior authorization formats. The precise form varies, but it also is a structured interview conducted by the MCO/insurance company staff member. The MCO staff member may be a nurse or experienced mental health professional, or someone merely trained to do the interview. The interview may be based on a computerized decision tree or the MCO's staff member's personal interpretation of the clinical information. Some MCO/insurance reviewers get reputations of being unreasonable, rigorous, difficult, or unprofessional.[15,16] Furthermore, the MCO phone prior authorization may take as long as if not longer than the clinician's interview with the patient.

This section discusses completing the phone prior authorization. It covers a typical, expected outline for pre-certification. It also discusses strategies for challenging insurance reviewers.

As noted earlier, the phone prior authorization follows a structure. While the order varies, the clinician can expect the following questions:

- National Provider Identifier for the hospital
- National Provider Identifier for the physician
- Tax identification number for the hospital
- Patient's insurance identification number
- Type of admission: substance use/detox or mental health stabilization
- Reason for presentation
- Suicidal ideation
  - Plan?
  - When the patient last had a plan
  - Means and access to those means
  - Prior attempts
- Homicidal ideation
- Mental status
  - Affect and mood
  - Orientation to reality
  - Appearance/attendance to activities of daily living
  - Thought content (logical, disorganized, blocking, tangential, etc.)
  - Observed psychotic symptoms
- Substance use
  - Substances used
    - Amount
    - Route of use (intravenous, nasal, oral, smoking)
    - Frequency
  - Detox symptoms
    - Clinical Institute Withdrawal Assessment for Alcohol score
    - Clinical Opiate Withdrawal Scale score
    - Vital signs
  - Is the patient involved in recovery?
    - Alcoholics Anonymous
    - Narcotics Anonymous

Diagnosis

Diagnosis has not been discussed yet in this book. It matters the most in terms of prior authorization in classifying the reason for admission. The patient's primary diagnosis should match the reason for admission (i.e., mental health or detox). A diagnosis is essentially an organized classification of a patient's demonstrated, collective symptoms.

The standard for diagnoses is the *Diagnostic and Statistical Manual* (DSM) published by the American Psychiatric Association. At the time of writing, the current version of the DSM is the fifth version also known as DSM-5TR. The DSM-5TR utilizes the diagnostic codes of the International Classification of Diseases Tenth Revision,[17] which will be used in this book.

While the DSM-5 is a lengthy, complex book, it is recommended that the diagnosis either be an unspecified diagnosis versus a highly specified one. Examples of unspecified diagnoses include the following:

- F32.9 Major depressive disorder, single episode, unspecified[18]
- F29 Unspecified psychosis not due to a substance or known physiological condition
- F91.9 Conduct disorder, unspecified[19]

A reasonable exception is in the case of previous patients when the psychiatrist's documentation is available. The diagnosis from either the previous admitting psychiatric assessment or the discharge summary is appropriate to use in that the clinician is subscribing to a patient's documented clinical history.

In the case of substance use diagnoses, the clinician will usually need to choose from the following:[20]

- Alcohol use disorder (F10.xx)
- Opioid use disorder (F11.xx)
- Cannabis use disorder (F12.xx)
- Sedative, hypnotic, or anxiolytic-related use disorder (F13.xx)
- Cocaine use disorder (F14.xx)
- Amphetamine use disorder (F15.xx)
- Inhalant use disorder (F18.xx)
- Unspecified substance use disorder (F19.xx)

In all these diagnoses, the last two digits are used to signify the degree of severity.

- Mild use disorder is .10 in the last two spaces.
- Moderate to severe disorder is .20 in the last two spaces.[21]
- Medical conditions and whether the patient is medically clear.
- Medications and compliance.
- Known outpatient providers.
- Treatment history (if known).

As part of the prior authorization, the MCO may ask for some other organizational and treatment process questions that include

- contact numbers for the utilization review/management department,
- contact number for the discharge planner,
- treatment plan,[22]
- proposed discharge plan,
- how many treatment days are being requested,[23] and
- will best practices be used?[24]

The preferred answers to these questions should be part of the job orientation or in accessible reference material.

An MCO may have short forms and long forms of the interview that may be randomly implemented or based on the initial screening questions. The regular short form is a screening interview to save time and process prior authorizations quicker.

Regardless of the form, if the case is clear cut in the way of suicidal ideation, homicidal ideation, psychosis, or detox, the short form will be more likely used by the MCO and prior authorization will be granted regardless. If the case is not clear cut in the aforementioned ways or it is an out of control or highly aggressive child, then the clinician will likely be referred for the full review.

Strategies for Verbal Presentation and Possible Debate

As discussed earlier, the full phone review can be difficult. If it is not the questions, it can be MCO reviewers who are habitually argumentative with clinicians over the phone over any number of issues that seem irrelevant to the patient's case. In all fairness, insurance reviewers have standards that they must uphold and are accountable to their employers, and so they must challenge the clinician as to the validity of the assessment.[25] However, they too may be unhealthy professionals who have found that working in insurance is an escape (and possibly more lucrative work) from direct practice. Despite the likelihood of the conversation being recorded for training and quality assurance, the latter type of reviewer can be strangely critical and hostile in tone toward the clinician and even the patient whom they have not personally seen.[26]

There are several strategies for managing the phone prior authorization with the reviewer:

- Have the assessment (whether printed or on screen) in front of you.
- Let the reviewer lead the conversation.

- If the reviewer asks a question that is not part of the assessment, the clinician can say something to the effect of "The format of the assessment does not cover that question" or "We do not have the capability to do lab tests or drug screens in the department."
- Stay calm or at least practice modified boredom in your tone of voice.
- Ignore critical comments and personal attacks of your work and the patient.[27]
- Have your "arguments" ready, including
  - the main criteria/reason for admission and
  - supportive documentation to include risk factors to deflect reviewers who believe the case is weak or is simply a high utilizer or repeater patient.

The essential themes of dealing with a difficult reviewer are to be a mature and prepared professional who sticks to the facts and has emotional boundaries.

THE FAX AUTHORIZATION

At face value, the fax prior authorization is easier and time-saving but can lead to a critique of the clinician's thoroughness of assessment, logic, documentation, and penmanship and thus a denial due to poor quality. The clinician may not be made aware of this until after the fact and if there is a pattern of denials. Therefore, it is incumbent upon the clinician to create documentation that clearly communicates that the patient met criteria for admission.

The fax authorization typically consists of the submission of a worksheet and a paper copy of the clinician's assessment. The clinician will then transmit these documents to the MCO via a toll-free number.

Documentation quality can depend on the format used by the organization. The format may be typed, handwritten, or dictated by voice-recognition software. Each format has its challenges.

The typed assessment should be the most thorough and easiest to read, but it depends on the keyboarding skills of the clinician and can take the longest of the formats. This kind of assessment will be used in organizations that have invested in computerized medical recordkeeping and have made provision for it. The drawbacks include that not everyone has the same level of typing skill. Clinicians with lower levels of typing skill also gravitate to being concise, summarizing more (as opposed to quoting), and having more typographical errors, which means there is a risk that salient clinical details can be missed in the assessment.

The handwritten format assessment is usually a multi-page set of printed forms with lines and boxes. It tends to be used in proprietary psychiatric hospital systems that have paper-based documentation systems. Timewise, it is the most efficient of the assessment formats, but it depends on the quality and legibility of the clinician's penmanship.

Whether handwritten or typed, both formats typically have a clinical summary paragraph that is crucial to the prior authorization.[28] This paragraph should summarize the clinical data in a logical order and state a clinical recommendation as an outcome.

The order of the paragraph should be as follows:

- demographics (age, sex, race),[29]
- how seen (telehealth, walk-in, fax referral),
- chief complaint,
- citing of collateral sources,
- review of clinical symptoms and functioning ("activities of daily living"),
- review of suicidal and homicidal ideation status,
- existence or absence of psychosis,
- substance use,
- review of mental status,
- risk factors,
- possible precipitants of the problem, and
- review of patient with a physician or licensed provider and the outcome.

The length of the paragraph will vary based on how much needs to be explained. The clear-cut cases can be explained in short paragraphs while the patients who are "on the line" will require more explanation as to why inpatient admission is necessary. The following are some examples of summary paragraphs using these guidelines.

Example #1: The Suicidal Patient

The patient is a forty-three-year-old African American male who presented on a walk-in basis reporting suicidal ideation. The patient reported that he has been having thoughts of suicidal ideation today and yesterday with a plan of running out into traffic. The patient denied homicidal ideation and psychosis. The patient was oriented to reality times four and evidenced depressed affect. The patient reported that he drinks about five twelve-ounce beers a day and last drank about two days ago. The case was staffed with Dr. Johnson who accepted the patient for inpatient admission.

Example #2: The Homicidal Patient

The patient is a twenty-six-year-old Caucasian male who presented to Crosstown Hospital's emergency department and who was seen via telehealth. The patient reported having homicidal ideations with a plan to shoot his sister's boyfriend. The patient said that his sister was beaten by the boyfriend. The patient denied suicidal ideation and psychosis. The patient reported daily use of about one-half ounce of marijuana and two lines of meth. The patient reported last using marijuana yesterday and last using meth three days ago. Collateral information from a nurse at the emergency department included that the patient had a positive drug screen for cannabis, meth, and cocaine. The patient evidenced orientation to reality times four and labile affect. The case was staffed with Dr. Michaels, who accepted the patient for inpatient admission.

Example #3: The Psychotic Patient

The patient is a thirty-eight-year-old Caucasian female who presented on a walk-in basis with her sister. The patient's sister reported that the patient has been off her medication, not sleeping, not bathing, and exhibiting bizarre behaviors that include talking to people who are not there. During the assessment, the patient refused to answer questions about suicide and homicidal ideation. The patient was also observed as demonstrating paranoia with poor eye contact, but also responding to internal stimuli. The patient was not oriented to day and situation. The patient presented as disheveled and malodorous. The case was staffed with Dr. Miller, who accepted the patient for admission on a seventy-two-hour hold.

Example #4: The Alcohol Detox Patient

The patient is a forty-eight-year-old Caucasian female presenting as a walk-in requesting detox services. The patient reported drinking one pint of vodka daily for six months with the last drink today about two hours prior to coming into the hospital. The patient had a blood alcohol level of 0.08 upon arrival. The patient evidenced a Clinical Institute Withdrawal Assessment for Alcohol score of fourteen. The patient denied suicidal ideation and homicidal ideation but reported feeling hopeless and helpless. The patient also reported poor sleep and appetite. The patient was oriented times four. The patient evidenced depressed and irritable affect, disheveled appearance, and was malodorous with the smell of alcohol. The case was staffed with the patient's previous provider, Dr. Khan, who accepted the patient for admission.

Example #5: The Opioid Detox Patient

The patient is a thirty-three-year-old male who presented for opiate detox. The patient reported using 1.0 gram of heroin via intravenous route daily for the past month. The patient reported last use to be two hours prior to presentation. The patient evidenced a Clinical Opiate Withdrawal Scale score of fifteen. The patient vomited during the assessment. The patient reported suicidal ideation with no plan. The patient denied homicidal ideation and psychosis. The patient also reported daily use of cannabis and intravenous use of meth two or three times per week with last use two days ago. The case was staffed with the next provider on rotation, Dr. Macy, who accepted the patient for admission.

Example #6: The Out of Control Child

The patient is a thirteen-year-old male who was brought by his foster mother after several events today. Thc patient had hit another child (age five) in the foster home causing facial bruising and punched a hole in the wall. Also, per the foster mother, the patient was throwing hard objects at the foster mother and a third child in the home. The foster mother said that she cannot keep things safe in the home. The patient was initially refusing to speak in the interview, but away from the foster mother, the patient admitted to hitting the five-year-old because he was annoyed by her. The patient denied suicidal ideation, homicidal ideation, and psychosis, and was oriented to reality times four. The patient evidenced irritable and depressed affect. The patient reported feeling helpless and hopeless. The case was staffed with the next provider on rotation, Dr. Smith, who accepted the patient for inpatient admission.

Example #7: The High Utilizer

The patient is a fifty-five-year-old Caucasian female who had was discharged from this facility three days ago. The patient presented as a walk-in and reported that she was suicidal but denied a plan but said that she if she were not admitted she would go out and kill herself by whatever way possible. The patient reported that she had homicidal ideation but refused to say the name of her intended victim and the intended method. The patient reported poor sleep, appetite, hopelessness, and helplessness. The patient said that she was hearing voices and experiencing visual hallucinations but refused to go into detail. The patient said that she has not been on her medication for two weeks. The case was staffed with the previous provider, Dr. Hamilton, who recommended inpatient admission for safety.[30]

Example #8: The Amphetamine User with Psychosis

The patient is a thirty-four-year-old Caucasian male who presented to the emergency room for chest pains. The patient's drug screen was positive for cannabis, opiates, and amphetamines. The patient reported to the emergency department staff that he had been hearing voices earlier in the day and having suicidal ideation. In the interview, the patient presented as disorganized and tangential. The patient also was observed responding to internal stimuli at one point in the interview. The patient denied current suicidal ideation and homicidal ideation, but was not oriented to time. The patient said that he had not slept in two days. The patient said that he wanted to come into the hospital. The case was staffed with the next provider on rotation, Dr. Wheeler, who accepted the patient for admission.

Example #9: The Transgender Adult

The patient is a thirty-nine-year-old black male to female transgender individual who presented as a walk-in reporting suicidal ideation with a plan to jump off a bridge. The patient reported having constant thoughts of suicide. The patient denied homicidal ideation and psychosis. The patient was oriented times four. The patient reported daily use of crack cocaine and weekly use of meth. The patient's preferred pronouns are they/them and that they had not taken their medication in about one month. The case was staffed with the previous provider, Dr. Erickson, who accepted the patient for inpatient admission.

Example #10: The Transgender Adolescent

The patient is a thirteen-year-old white female to male transgender individual who was brought by their mother due to suicidal ideation and out of control behavior. The patient had reported suicidal ideation with a plan to cut themselves. The patient denied homicidal ideation and psychosis. The patient was oriented to reality times four. It is noted that the mother made a statement of opposition to the patient's transgender status during the interview. The patient reported having tried vaping but denied any other substance use. The case was staffed with the next provider on rotation, Dr. Cupp, who accepted the patient for inpatient.

THE ONLINE AUTHORIZATION

The use of the online prior authorization varies by MCO and hospital. Not all MCOs offer online authorization and not all hospitals get access. If access is obtained by the hospital, it is an online form where the clinician briefly enters the case information as discussed in the fax authorization section and gets some kind of acknowledgment via reference or authorization number. This is a quick means of prior authorization but access to it is primarily the reason it is not utilized as much.

THE PEER-TO-PEER OR PHYSICIAN REVIEW

One potential outcome of the phone prior authorization encounter is a referral for a peer-to-peer review with a physician. The peer-to-peer review happens more so in prior authorization requests for cases that are "on the line" that do not clearly meet criteria. MCOs can also call for peer-to-peer reviews in the cases of high utilizers and out of control/aggressive children.[31] Insurance and MCOs have contracted physicians as on-call experts to conduct such peer reviews to ensure admissions and continued stay are both necessary and appropriate.

Logically, the immediate peer-to-peer review at the time of prior authorization can only be validly conducted in an emergency room of an academic hospital with a psychiatric unit that is staffed twenty-four hours a day with a resident who follows up the master's level clinician's work with their own assessment. In the context of this book where a master's level clinician is doing the assessment and the physician is only accepting the patient via a telephone staffing, it is unreasonable for the accepting physician to do a peer-to-peer review for a patient they have not seen yet.

Nevertheless, in the cases of requesting a peer-to-peer review when the physician is unavailable, the MCO may either issue a denial for prior authorization or suspend approval until it is completed. It is important for the clinician to be familiar with the hospital's policy for responding to the MCO's request for a peer-to-peer request in such cases.

WHAT IF THERE IS A DENIAL?

One of the inherent purposes of this book is to educate a clinician to get a prior authorization approval every time, but the reality is that despite careful assessment and acceptance by a provider, numerous admissions are going to be on the line and get denied. While the denials can help a clinician refine their skills over time, this type of practice setting is more about erring on the side of safety than letting a potentially unsafe patient (who wants to be admitted) leave and perhaps go complete suicide or kill someone. A denial does not mean that the clinician has done a poor job of assessing the patient, nor has the clinician failed at making an appropriate treatment recommendation.

There are multiple reasons for denials beyond the dispute of an admission being appropriate and necessary. MCOs can change their standards or practices or add a new requirement without notice. An MCO reviewer can act in a rogue or erratic fashion and say they are not going to grant the prior authorization. A patient who has a managed Medicare may have used all their 180, lifetime, psychiatric inpatient days and receive a "technical denial." Dealing with insurance denials should be part of the job orientation and training process, and the clinician should discuss with their supervisors about how to handle such situations, especially when MCOs change their prior authorization practices.

CONCLUDING THOUGHTS

Assessment clinicians in the United States will likely have to master the prior authorization process. Prior authorization is the beginning phase of utilization management process where the MCO or payor source makes initial approval of an admission.

The manner and rigor of prior authorization depends on the payor source, and it can change from time to time. Even if it is a Medicaid patient, MCOs tend to be for-profit organizations who have a vested interest in saving the government money so as to improve their bottom lines, and so, prior authorizations can become tougher to screen out more admissions to be unnecessary and inappropriate. Even in clear-cut cases, MCOs may conduct a time-consuming and rigorous prior authorization that asks for all kinds of details, only to approve one per day for all the clinician's work.

Overall, a prior authorization is predictable. It has a generally predictable order as discussed in this chapter and the organized, prepared clinician can successfully navigate it.

Difficulty in the phone prior authorization can be had when an MCO has reviewers who have difficult personalities, less than professional tones of voice, argumentative styles, and act with low emotional intelligence that comes across as inappropriate judgmental or derogatory comments about the patient. What is supposed to be a professional encounter can erupt into an emotional argument which interferes with the clinician's completion of the job. In these regrettable situations, it is incumbent on the clinician to remain calm with such reviewers as they were with the patients.

The fax prior authorization circumvents dealing with a live MCO reviewer and the potential arguments, but it does require the clinician to compose an orderly, clinical summary. The effective clinical summary has predictive elements that were addressed in this chapter.

There will be occasional denials despite how thorough the clinician was with the assessment and smooth in demonstrating that criteria for admission was met to an MCO reviewer. The reality is that there is an aspect of gamesmanship in the relationship between providers, MCOs, and the insurance industry; the latter will change standards and practices without notice that show up in prior authorization encounters.

For the assessment clinician who perseveres, the matter of prior authorization can make them better. To know a patient's insurance prior to the interview gives a clinician a sense of the rigor and peculiarities ahead to ask the additional questions to establish whether criteria for admission has been met. However, prior authorizations by phone are truly part of the growth and development process for a clinician as much as mastering the assessment process.

NOTES

1. Different carriers have different terms that all refer to the same concept of getting approval for the admission at the time of admission. "InterQual" has historically used the term "initial review" throughout its volumes. Another term is "prospective review," but the term "prior authorization" will be used here given its prevalence in the literature.
2. In Canada, hospital admission is not subject to prior authorization like in the United States.
3. For the most part in the United States, the state and federal governments have privatized utilization management by contracting it out to MCOs, insurance companies, and fiscal intermediaries. Much of the time the MCOs are insurance companies themselves. Some MCOs are insurance company subcontractors. However, there are a few MCO exceptions like Kaiser Permanente and Mayo Clinic that are not insurance companies.
4. In the experience of the authors, one MCO has switched back and forth between phone calls and faxes.
5. Some prior authorizations can qualify for short forms based on the answer to a few key indicating questions including that the patient is clearly suicidal or detoxing. Some MCOs have a random approach of long form versus short form prior authorizations.
6. The reviewer will usually read some disclaimer at the end of a prior authorization phone call that payment is not guaranteed. It will be dependent on the demonstration of the course of treatment.
7. J. A. Mitus, 2008, "The birth of InterQual: Evidence-based decision support criteria that helped change healthcare," *Professional Case Management, 13*(4): 228–33.
8. Internationally, countries with "socialized" medicine that consist of totally government-funded healthcare systems have engaged in forms of utilization review to manage the inherently limited funding available.
9. S. Daniels and R. L. Hirsch, 2015, *The hospital guide to contemporary utilization review*, Danvers, MA: HCPro.
10. A different definition by Montgomery (2021) is that utilization review is the process of making sure healthcare services are being used appropriately and efficiently. Its goal is to make sure patients get the care they need, that it is administered

via proven methods, provided by an appropriate healthcare provider, and delivered in an appropriate setting. K. Montgomery, 2021, "Benefits of a value-based payment system," *verywellhealth*, https://www.verywellhealth.com/what-is-pay-for-performance-1738536.

11. In 2010, there was a trend toward both utilization management and retrospective utilization review by Medicare fiscal intermediaries that involved incentivized auditors.

12. Medicaid is a jointly funded program; both the states and the federal government contribute to it. Different US states had various forms of Medicaid utilization review that was referred to as "capitation" or a ceiling of funds.

13. Hospitals have utilization management departments to oversee the management of care and to interact with MCOs, insurance companies, and designated government agencies to get reimbursed.

14. If the case is denied, the provider either must discharge the patient or absorb the cost and appeal the denial.

15. The prior authorization is a very human process. The MCOs have goals and standards themselves and the reviewers themselves are accountable for the interview.

16. MCO reviewers also have different levels of clinical competence. For example, in the author's personal experience, while doing a prior authorization on a ten-year-old, the reviewer asked if the patient was involved in Alcoholics Anonymous. This reviewer had the reputation of asking every question on the script for every prior authorization regardless of whether it was irrelevant to the type of patient.

17. The International Classification of Diseases is maintained by the World Health Organization.

18. American Psychiatric Association, 2022, *Diagnostic and statistical manual of mental disorders* (fifth edition), Washington, DC: American Psychiatric Association.

19. American Psychiatric Association, 2022, *Diagnostic and statistical manual of mental disorders* (fifth edition), Washington, DC: American Psychiatric Association, 530–39. Within this type of assessment, determination of onset of conduct disorder is not necessary.

20. These are common diagnoses that the clinician can encounter. American Psychiatric Association, 2022, *Diagnostic and statistical manual of mental disorders* (fifth edition), Washington, DC: American Psychiatric Association, 553–651.

21. The determination of substance use severity level is a judgment call for the clinician, but it is suggested by the number of symptoms the patient has: two to three for mild, four to five for moderate, and six or more for severe. American Psychiatric Association, 2022, *Diagnostic and statistical manual of mental disorders* (fifth edition), Washington, DC: American Psychiatric Association, 554. However, in cases where the patient may be coming in with amphetamine-induced psychosis (F15.259), it would be logical that the patient also would have a diagnosis of F15.20, amphetamine use disorder, severe.

22. An answer to this question could go something like this: medication management, safety checks every fifteen minutes, group therapy, milieu therapy, individual therapy, and possible family therapy.

23. Sometimes this is a moot question because the number of days approved is according to the computer algorithm used by the MCO or MCO policies, but a good practice is to ask for three to four days. Some organizations may have a policy to ask for seven days.

24. The clinician's answer should be "Yes."

25. The phone call with the reviewer may have a third party listening in on the conversation or it may be recorded.

26. See D. Houvenagle, 2015, *Clinician's guide to partial hospitalization and intensive outpatient practice*, New York: Springer Publishing Company, chapter 16.

27. Ignoring for this purpose is not reacting or even responding to personal attacks and maybe even playing silent.

28. The summary paragraph also matters when referring the patient to another psychiatric hospital.

29. There may be a question as to the extent of demographic description that is required. In this context, discussion of the patient's gender identity in addition to biological sex is only clinically relevant for placement purposes. Most facilities only require identification if a patient is transgender for determination of bed availability. While it is a demonstration of a clinician's political correctness or adherence to diversity, equity, and inclusion practice, discussion of a patient's sexual orientation and use of the term *cisgender* in summaries only adds irrelevant wordiness unless it is clinically relevant to the patient's primary complaint.

30. With the high utilizer, the clinician must be thorough and more detailed in the summary paragraph. The clinician often must reverse the thought process, looking for every valid reason for not admitting the patient. Some high utilizers can present as entitled, indignant, and intimidating where they give as little detail as possible. On the other hand, other high utilizers present as "dumb" or ignorant that suggests the assumption of they do not remember being in the hospital even though they were just there. A third category of high utilizer gives precisely the necessary information to get into the hospital. If the clinician has access to the digital medical record, there likely will be information that contradicts the patient's claims about when they were last on medication.

31. The MCO contracted physician is typically in another state. The degree of physician involvement varies from MCO to MCO, and it has varied over time as MCOs have changed their decision trees. Some MCOs may require the reviewer to call and review in turn with the physician or request the peer-to-peer review.

Chapter 13

The High Utilizer

The average assessment clinician will have to interview a high utilizer. These individuals are pejoratively called frequent flyers or rapid readmitters. Both terms refer to an adult individual who frequently presents to a hospital emergency department with some kind of complaint or to an intake department of a psychiatric hospital. There is no discernible consensus as to a standard frequency of admission for a patient to be labeled a high utilizer. Furthermore, there are no discernible accepted methods for interviewing a high utilizer, but many of the earlier vignettes in the book have arisen out of the experience of the authors with this type of patient.

The matter of high utilizers is not restricted to the United States. International research has shown that up to 13 percent of psychiatric patients are readmitted within ninety days of discharge. High utilizers have a sustained pattern of rapid readmissions. The matter of high utilizers is of interest to both researchers and policy makers so as to reduce healthcare costs, and there are numerous academic articles that seek to understand this population and create strategies to reduce readmissions.[1]

High utilizers are a complex group with diverse clinical and psychosocial factors, but they have some similar behaviors. They demonstrate savviness in saying the right things to meet admission criteria on a repetitive basis. This savviness includes cooperating as little as possible with the interview, instigating disruptive drama, and being threatening in the department. Many nascent clinicians have been shaken by the experience of dealing with the high utilizer. What is more, it is the experience of the authors that upon admission to the hospital that many high utilizers prove to be malingers who are non-compliant with both treatment and discharge planning, yet claim continency-based suicidal ideation when it is time to go (I am going to go kill myself if you discharge me). For all intents and purposes, profiling high utilizers serves as a framework for understanding, maintaining a professional attitude, conducting an effective interview, and properly documenting the assessment.

This chapter explores the matter of the high utilizer as well as clinical skills and strategies for completing assessments with this type of patient based on the experiences of the authors. Typically, if a high utilizer presents again after such a short time (from the day of discharge to one week), it requires meticulousness and detailed reporting on the clinician's part to provide valid and substantial criteria to get a successful prior authorization. However, many high utilizers are uncooperative with the clinician's need to be meticulous in the interview, leading to both frustration and countertransference. If the clinician must interview the same high utilizer repetitively, the onus is upon the clinician to maintain consistent professionalism considering the practical reality of developing countertransference. The clinician has both emotional and professional challenges in interviewing this patient.

DESCRIBING HIGH UTILIZERS

The matter of describing a high utilizer patient is complex as there are multiple clinical and psychosocial factors. While there are children and adolescents who could be identified as high utilizers due to the frequency of readmission and long stays, the focus in the available literature is on adults as the primary clinical factors are diagnoses of schizophrenia and a personality disorder.[2] Other clinical factors include suicidal ideation.[3] Some high utilizers also have lower intellectual functioning. Social factors of high utilization include poverty, medical complexity, housing instability, and substance use.[4] The most prevalent demographic is non-Hispanic white females between the ages of forty-six to fifty-four.[5] Drug addiction and oppressing factors of homelessness may have degenerative effects on a person's motivation, problem-solving skills, and self-concept that manifest as a regression in functioning or exacerbation of psychiatric symptoms. It is difficult to write a proposition that encompasses the high utilizer in terms of the whole admission and discharge process, but it is safe to say that the high utilizer in general fails to follow through with outpatient aftercare in one manner or another and readmits rapidly.

Figure 13.1 is a simplified, graphical conception of the variations of psychiatric high utilizers. Most high utilizers tend to have a variable combination of true mental illness, substance use, and personality disorder. However, there are high utilizers who are schizophrenic without substance use and personality disorder. There are high utilizers who present as having purely substance use issues with frequent relapse. And there are high utilizers who present as

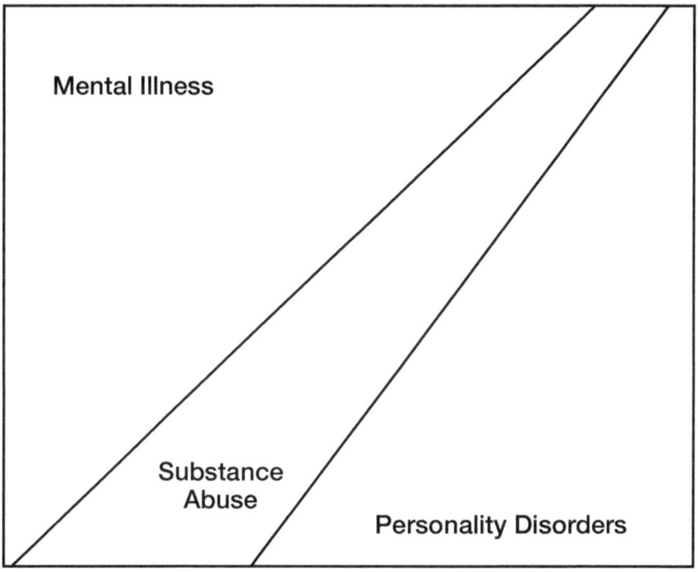

Figure 13.1. Variations in Presentations of High Utilizers.

purely demonstrating personality disorders. Many high utilizers can vary in their symptom complaint at different presentations where one time they are suicidal, another time they are predominantly detoxing, and a third time they are experiencing severe psychosis.

Symptoms aside, when reading Maslow's Hierarchy of Needs, high utilizers indeed present as having problems meeting the first two levels of physiological and safety needs. High utilizers often have limited viable to absolutely no family support.[6] Furthermore, many patients are "institutionalized" or institutionally dependent and while they seem to have verbal skills to suggest the necessary executive functioning, they lack the motivation/ego skills to demonstrate self-sufficiency in independently structuring their lives and consistently meeting their physical, social, and emotional needs. Many high utilizers seem to fit the picture of the underclass put forth by Wilson[7] of being unable to function independently in society and likely are "transinstitutionalized" or going to whatever societal institution can care for them, which if it is not the hospital, then the relevant correctional facility.[8] In large part because they cannot meet safety needs, high utilizers are logically exposed to trauma situations, and thus have some trauma-related impairments, and deserve some empathetic, trauma-informed care approaches.

However, the empathy regarding trauma exposure can frequently dry up because many high utilizers evidence to be malingerers with pathological traits, whose claims of suicidal ideation or other symptoms manifest as being for secondary gains such as homelessness or avoidance of legal obligations (court dates, appointments with probation parole, required drug screens).[9,10] Dealing with them can be stressful as they are either passive-aggressive or openly hostile toward inpatient staff as opposed to taking responsibility for problem solving.

When eventually admitted, it has been the experience of the authors that typical high utilizers also are difficult to engage in both treatment and discharge planning to stop the cycle of rapid readmissions. They tend to evidence one or more of the following:

- treatment savviness and manipulative behaviors toward unit staff,[11]
- minimal involvement in treatment groups,
- withdrawal from the therapeutic milieu by staying in their beds, and
- uncooperativeness if not "gaminess" with social workers in discharge planning.

The unit behavior clearly reflects the demographic traits discussed here, and it connects with the patient's inability to cooperate with social work efforts.[12]

The lack of compliance with social work and discharge planning seems to be reflective of the patient personality traits and the lack of resources. High utilizers also have a high likelihood of

- losing discharge papers,
- missing outpatient appointments (if not readmitted before them),
- not getting prescriptions filled (if they did not lose the paper scripts first), and
- failure at lower levels of care that include rehab.

Many high utilizers do not evidence the ego strength or executive functioning found in the average person to show responsibility to follow through with aftercare. What is more, for any patient (and not just the high utilizer) to make the necessary aftercare changes that would help them maintain stability at the outpatient level, they usually need some kind of housing and security resources (Maslow's first level of needs).

There is a variant of high utilizer where the patient has a valid diagnosis of schizophrenia or bipolar disorder with a true presentation of psychosis. This kind of high utilizer does not want to take their medications but is compelled to come back to the hospital whenever they are in a mental health crisis because of the return of symptoms. This category of high utilizer could be said to have co-occurring disorders or dual diagnosis, where they prefer to self-medicate with illicit substances and manifest addiction symptoms, and they are not considered to be good candidates for residential rehab due to the overall severe and persistent mental illness. This type of high utilizer is in a discernible cycle where they are not malingering but are also not motivated to change.

High utilizers who occasionally have a successful discharge plan to include a substance use rehab or a group home typically return after a relatively short period of time given the inability to cope, comply, or function in that setting (see the comment about hypersensitivity in the following). A high utilizer with drug addiction either has significant personality disorder issues and the inherent lack of ego strength to handle the emotional stress and strain of rehab and/or is ambivalent about recovery.[13] The high utilizer that disrupts an adult group home placement typically has the inability to submit to the order and rules of such settings in addition to problems getting along with other residents and not being in control of their disability payments. It is often a matter of time before a high utilizer has exhausted reasonable discharge resources due to their behaviors as part of the cycle of readmission.

High utilizers with personality disorders demonstrate emotional hypersensitivity as part of the lack of ego strength and do not evidence normal coping patterns which can make meaningful participation in drug rehab facilities impossible. Talking about their problems with a stranger can ironically be the infliction of emotional pain for the high utilizer. Psychoanalytically, they have ego deficits and cannot handle what they existentially view as pain and demonstrate avoidance that may be passive aggressiveness toward the clinician and others. If not being avoidant, there is the likelihood of their instigation of drama by portraying themselves as victims through making claims of being offended or hurt by making some of the following passionate comments:

- They talked to me like I was a dog (or a piece of sh-t).
- Please do not yell at me (when confronted in a normal speaking voice).
- Are you mad at me? I just cannot handle people being mad at me.
- I was disrespected.

The manner in which they make these claims can vary from a position of self-righteous anger or from a desperate sounding victim (which is the potential instigation of drama).

If the high utilizer does not play the victim, they often demonstrate control issues especially when they collect social security or disability payments. Some high utilizers with disability, who could be referred to group homes, have no interest in giving up control of their money to pay for those room and board expenses.[14] Some of the resistance to commit to group homes may be purely be out of control needs, or it may be related to the high utilizer's addiction.

Depending on the situation, it can appear that the psychiatrist who continues to readmit a high utilizer is enabling the patient.[15] Nevertheless, previous doctors often feel pressured to readmit high utilizers or they will lose the patients off their caseload. Given the previous comments about treatment non-compliance, the high utilizer is a frustrating patient to deal with for multiple hospital employees at different organizational levels and at different stages in the treatment process.

Many high utilizers can stay in the hospital for lengthy periods through the claim of contingency-based suicidal ideation. They increase their suicidal statements, and they may even make a threat to kill themselves if they are discharged.[16] The eventual discharge is contingent upon the doctor's tolerance of risk, the treatment team's determination that treatment benefit has been maximized, or the patient's request to leave for whatever personal reasons.

Some high utilizers move from hospital to hospital in a circuit.[17] In the experience of the authors, the circuit is more likely to be within the same metropolitan area, but some have amazingly demonstrated mobility through managing to get admitted in distant hospitals in a rapid manner. Also, anecdotally, some high utilizers have been discharged from a hospital in one city and presented at another hospital in a distant city within one day. In these cases, the high utilizer frequently tells a perfidious story to the next assessment clinician that excludes the detail that they were just discharged from another hospital; at face value, it usually appears that they have been out of the hospital for an extended period, have not had their medications for an extended period, and are meeting criteria for admission. The only ways the assessment clinician learns about the fact of the high utilizer's recent discharge from another hospital is if an insurance reviewer discloses it during a live review for a prior authorization or they happen to talk with the previous hospital.[18]

In a practical sense, if an insurance reviewer issues a denial on a high utilizer due to a recent admission, the clinician should consult their supervisor for current policy. There are varying policies for such situations. The hospital may appeal the denial and/or the doctor may discharge the patient the next day after a face-to-face assessment.

In the experience of the authors, the primary ways in which high utilizers have not been readmitted are that the high utilizer died, the high utilizer was incarcerated for a criminal offense and in a correctional facility, or the high utilizer was administratively restricted from further admission. Regardless of the analysis, the high utilizer presents again and again with a subjective claim of clinical symptomology that will make them meet criteria for admission.[19] The clinician may have to interview the same high utilizers repeatedly with all the potential countertransference and pressure.

OVERALL PERSPECTIVE

Reducing or halting the admissions of the high utilizers verbalizing symptoms (suicidal ideation, homicidal ideation, severe psychosis) that meets the criteria of immediate safety risk is not going to be in the hands of the assessment clinician. As discussed earlier in the book, the master's level clinician should not outrightly try to restrict a high utilizer from being admitted to a hospital out of the view that a patient is merely malingering when reporting symptoms that meet criteria.[20] The clinician should never take that risk alone, and only do so if there is patient-specific direction from the administration.[21] Restricting high utilizers from further admission is largely a political and economic matter in the hands of administrators and policy makers. Especially with regards to the high utilizer, the space that the assessment clinician operates in is bureaucratic in its narrowness.

A hospital's organizational policy on high utilizers is not always clear but the suggestions given here are manifested based on a hospital's position in the marketplace as well as the patient's point of entry in the system. A proprietary hospital unattached to a medical hospital, but that has contracted to provide assessments at medical-surgical emergency rooms, has the tendency to defer high utilizers to nonprofit or public hospitals (this is especially true if the high utilizer has used all 180 lifetime Medicare behavioral health days).[22] Proprietary hospitals also may directly refer high utilizers to other facilities even if the patients are on their property for any number of behavioral reasons. Furthermore, while it seems that a psychiatrist is enabling a high utilizer by repeated readmissions, if the provider refuses to accept, the clinician may be compelled by a supervisor or informal policy to go to the next provider on rotation to admit a patient regardless out of concerns for liability and risk management. So many providers will continue to readmit high utilizers due to hospital policy.

SERIAL BEHAVIORAL PATTERNS

Getting back to the admitting phase, it is the experience of the authors that many (but not all) high utilizers demonstrate serial patterns of behavioral escalation for the purpose of manipulation. One escalation pattern is that the patient threatens or exhibits aggressive behavior shortly after assessment that necessitates crisis team escort to the unit in the name of safety; it is a way to manipulate getting to the unit faster and avoid waiting for hours to get to their bed.[23] A second pattern is when the high utilizer comes into the admitting department waiting room and physically acts out before the interview that necessitates restraint or seclusion. (The patient is often intoxicated or under the influence of drugs in these cases.) A third pattern is a combination of the high utilizer's detailed knowledge of department resources and sense of entitlement when they demand an item that they know the admitting or emergency department usually stocks (food, recliner, blanket) and if they do not get it immediately, they act out.[24] A possible answer for such disruptive behavior is related to the ego deficit of the patient. Whether the patient truly has a purpose for the behavior (as discussed in chapter 6) is not always discernable, but it is a way that high utilizers circumvent the order of the process, often presenting a challenge for the clinician to complete a satisfactory assessment document to get a prior authorization.

CHALLENGES TO INTERVIEWING

Given the serial behaviors, the clinician must interview (or at least attempt to interview) the high utilizer to establish whether the immediate safety risk criteria are met. Furthermore, the clinician should focus on conducting a valid, objective interview that specifies what has happened within the time frame between the known last date of discharge and the current assessment. The clinician has several challenges in this.

The first challenge is that within the patient's place on the curve of ability (discussed in chapters 3 and 6), the clinician must establish admission criteria to get a successful prior authorization. The high utilizer may be genuinely intoxicated and cognitively impaired. Otherwise, the treatment savviness of many high utilizers is manifested by their experience and knowledge of both the assessment and admission processes; they have been through the interview and know the questions—especially the ones they do not want to answer. With repetitive admissions, they have developed an appreciation of the minimum that must be said and what must be said (and how it must be said) to get admitted (see chapter 3, vignette #3). This appreciation also includes the knowledge of how to avoid those subjects they want to avoid.

Furthermore, as part of saying the minimum, some high utilizers will state what the admitting criteria is (even in the clinical jargon), and then avoid going through the whole interview by refusing to talk further, pretending to be asleep, or abruptly walking out of the room.[25] They frequently refuse to answer any further questions in an agitated and aggressive manner, with an excuse that they are in detox or that they do not feel good. Essentially, this is a power move on the patient's part as it usually leaves the clinician with numerous blanks on the interview that are expected to be filled, and it can leave the newer clinician in a somewhat desperate situation.

The second challenge is both emotional and professional for the clinician in managing countertransference and emotional boundaries with the patient.

Some high utilizers with personality disorders blatantly antagonize clinicians in ways that amount to bullying of newer clinicians. They can make personal attacks on the clinician or claim to be personally offended by the interview questions despite having answered them before. As a human being, the clinician can experience the anger variations of disgust, annoyance, and frustration given the challenge of dealing with the patient, especially when such a patient tries to "arm-chair quarterback" (They did not ask this the last time!) or tries to intimidate the newer clinician in various ways (IS THIS ALMOST DONE?) to participate as minimally as possible. The newer clinician may also feel negative emotions of anxiety and embarrassment in reaction to the patient's anger.[26] However, the clinician must stay in the rational frame of mind and focus not to react emotionally to the personal attacks; the clinician must mindfully remain the adult in the room. The reader is referred to chapter 6 and the techniques of modified boredom and paradoxical affirmation of emotion.

The third challenge is to understand your organization's policies and philosophies on dealing with high utilizers. There may not be a codified policy in the book or organizational online database; however, there may be a set of directives that are easily ascertained with a series of questions to supervisors, managers, and directors.

STRATEGIES FOR INTERVIEWING DIFFICULT HIGH UTILIZERS

In accordance with these challenges, the following are some strategies for interviewing difficult high utilizers who have histories of minimal cooperation to maximize the information obtained. These strategies include

- using the quickest mode possible,
- entering known demographic and known history questions prior to the interview,
- establishing immediate safety risk and then working toward other subjects, and
- asking as many confirming questions as possible as opposed to open-ended questions.

These pragmatic strategies are based on the experience of the authors from actual interviews.

Use the Quickest Mode of Interviewing as Possible

As discussed in chapter 2, the typical interview is structured and ordered in the name of reliability. If the organization is using a computer form with a backup paper copy when the system is down, it would be best to use the latter. The computer version is slower, and many high utilizers are impatient and uncooperative with the order of the interview and the time that it takes to get through it.

Pre-Enter Demographic Information and Known History Prior to the Interview

When possible, entering or writing down the high utilizer's historical and demographic information can assist in speeding the interview along. Such information categories include

- educational attainment,
- previous suicide ideation history,
- developmental history,
- medical procedure history,
- ages of first use of the different drug classes,
- detox symptom history, and
- treatment history.

The historical categories are typically unchanged. The high utilizer also has had more admissions than allowed for in either the paper or computer forms. Furthermore, the clinician can build on the high utilizer's recent substance use and medical procedures, as will be discussed later.

Establish Immediate Safety Risk First

The clinician should first establish the high utilizer's immediate safety risk. Unless intoxicated to the point of anesthesia, the savvy high utilizer tends to take care of this by blurting that they had suicidal ideation with a plan or that they had tried to kill themselves on the day that they presented before they try to end the session. After reviewing the presenting problem, suicidal ideation, homicidal ideation, and psychosis, the clinician should consider going in the following order in terms of categories:

- mental status,
- substance use,
- last compliance with medications,
- other depressive symptoms,
    - sleep
    - appetite
    - activities of daily living (bathing)
    - hopelessness/helplessness

- new medical issues,
- sexual history,
- abuse history, and
- social support.

Ask Confirming Questions on History

Starting with the substance use questions, it can be helpful to ask questions in a confirmatory fashion. Examples of this include the following:

- When was the last time you drank alcohol?
- We know you started using marijuana at eighteen. When was the last time you used it?
- Since you were last here, have you used ___________ (name of substance)?
- We know you have blood pressure issues; do you have any other new medical problems?
- I know that you were discharged on Seroquel, Prozac, and Buspar; when was the last time you took your meds?
- From previous history, you were sexually, physically, and emotionally abused. Is there any new abuse or recent trauma you wish to report?

With this approach, some high utilizers will contradict previous disclosures about drug use or trauma. Such contradictions should be noted, but the previous information should be left in the assessment, as it was likely accurate that the high utilizer previously said it in the first place.

Set Soft Limits When the Patient Pushes to End the Interview Early

Some high utilizers who are repeatedly non-compliant with the interview will leave the room, stop talking, or be hostile and possibly threatening toward the clinician to end the interview. However, some high utilizers may try to end the interview by making statements of annoyance or agitation like in vignette #1 of chapter 4 where they essentially try to intimidate and gaslight the clinician.[27]

Again, using a tone of modified boredom and scripts of assertiveness, the clinician should set soft limits with the high utilizer. Some of the limits may be brief assertive statements. Other statements of limit may have to be empathetically and educational, as illustrated in vignette #1. There is no guarantee that the clinician is going to keep the high utilizer in the room for all the questions.

SOMETIMES YOU CAN DIVERT THE HIGH UTILIZER

One motivating reason a high utilizer has for repetitively seeking admission is to avoid homelessness and sleeping on the street. However, providing psychoeducation and having resources prepared to offer them allows a clinician to defer each patient to the appropriate resource. There are two strategies that a clinician can utilize to divert the high utilizer in an ethical manner.

The first strategy is, prior to starting a high utilizer's assessment, communicating the services the hospital provides upon doctor referral, and that they can be provided with information about community resources such as homeless shelters, case management, transportation, medical office contacts, etc. This will hopefully put it in the individual's head that their issue can be resolved by options other than psychiatric hospital admission.

The second strategy is a conversation the clinician can have with the high utilizer post assessment. It should be implemented when both A and B are true:

A. The high utilizer did not disclose any criteria warranting admission (suicidality, homicidal ideation, acute psychosis, erratic behavior, acute drug/alcohol withdrawal) during the assessment. The individual will, therefore, be referred to outpatient treatment.
B. The high utilizer is likely to "up the ante" when they are being referred to outpatient treatment. They will likely respond to the referral with something like, "What?! Outpatient?! What do you mean?! No, I need to be admitted. Fine. I am suicidal. Call my doctor and tell him that!"

The clinician should present resources tailored to the high utilizer's needs to couple the referral to outpatient treatment. In the same breath the clinician presents the outpatient referral, the clinician provides tailored referral forms that address the patient's needs for shelter, food, medical services, transportation, etc. There is a chance that this will preempt their immediate concerns of the following:

- Where will I stay and eat?
- How will I get to the outpatient program without a car?
- What about my insulin dosages needing to be adjusted?

It is the extent and desperation of these immediate concerns that likely influence many high utilizers to panic and endorse suicidality to get admitted.

If prior to the assessment the high utilizer blurts out, "I'm suicidal!" or reports any admittable criteria during the assessment (suicidal, homicidal, acute psychosis, erratic behavior, acute drug/alcohol withdrawal) then the clinician should not attempt to sway them into recanting or convince them that they do not need to be admitted. It is a liability and safety risk for the clinician to 1) talk a suicidal patient out of admission on the presumption they are manipulating the system, and 2) to trigger patient hostility by suggesting they are lying just to be admitted.

VIGNETTES

The following are two vignettes of interviewing high utilizers. The first vignette is from the previous section in diverting a high utilizer. The second vignette depicts the technique of maximizing the information when the high utilizer has a history of being non-compliant or only partially compliant with the assessment interview.

Vignette #1: Deferring the High Utilizer

Sebastian is a forty-three-year-old male who has averaged three admissions per month at the same hospital for the past four years. There have been occasions where he has been discharged out the front door of the hospital, only to walk around the back to get assessed and readmitted the same day. Sebastian's Medicaid managed care organization has been hesitant to grant coverage for more than a single day stay at the hospital due to his numerous hospitalizations. Each time he is assessed, he reports feeling suicidal from "everything." However, Sebastian frequently emphasizes that he cannot endure sleeping outside anymore and that he just wants to kill himself when he is alone in the alley or park. Rick, the assessment clinician, was familiar with Sebastian and hoped to defer readmission. Prior to the assessment, Rick reviewed Sebastian's previous assessments and prepared to talk with Sebastian about his physical needs prior to their clinical assessment and identify specific resources to meet Sebastian's needs.

Clinician: Hi Sebastian. My name is Rick, and I'll be completing your assessment today.

Sebastian: That's fine.

Clinician: Before we get started, I want to let you know about all our department can offer you in terms of treatment and social support. As you know, we offer psychiatric care on an inpatient and outpatient basis but we also help people get set up with case management to address housing, medical care, transportation, and nutrition. We also get people connected with homeless shelters, halfway houses, medical emergency departments/hospitals, soup kitchens, and community support networks. We can offer you a bus pass or taxi to your next destination if it is not with us and the back and forth commute if you are referred outpatient for treatment.

Sebastian: Case management? Where I get that?

Clinician: Have you heard of Center Rock? They have three offices in a five-mile radius and are open six days a week. I can make sure to contact them after the assessment to schedule you an appointment, if you would like.

Sebastian: That'd be dope.

Clinician: Yeah. I think you could really benefit from their services and your insurance entitles you to it!

Sebastian: That's what's up! Y'all get me to a shelter place tonight?

Clinician: Yes sir. I can call to reserve you a space after the assessment and then we'll work on getting you a bus pass or cab voucher.

Sebastian: Right on. So, do I go back to the waiting room now?

Clinician: Not yet sir. Let's complete an assessment together and see if you might be eligible for any of our services as well.

Sebastian: Cool doc. You know you alright. No one really talked to me about all that stuff available.

Clinician: I'm glad to make you aware of all your options.

Vignette #2: A High Utilizer with Personality Disorder and Substance Use

Violet is a forty-nine-year-old female who had fifteen previous admissions in the past six months. She presented for admission again after being discharged four days ago. Violet is known for being disruptive and rude to staff and other patients in the admitting waiting room. She appeared to be intoxicated on this presentation and prior to her turn had yelled repeatedly at staff because she had to wait for a blanket and a sack lunch, and because she was having to wait to be interviewed.

The clinician who drew Violet's name saw that she barely filled out her demographic form. The clinician reviewed her two previous assessments in the system and then grabbed a paper copy of the assessment normally used for times when the computer system is down and filled in Violet's

- demographics,
- trauma history,

- substance use history,
- medical history, and
- history of previous suicidal ideation and attempts.

The clinician called Violet into the interview room and got her vitals and blood alcohol level (which was a 0.10). After the preparation and getting her vitals, the clinician started the interview.

Clinician: Ms. Violet, I am sure you know me, I'm Dave and I'm going to do your interview as fast as I can. What brought you back here?

Violet: I tried to kill myself today by walking out into traffic.

Clinician: Was there anything else that happened since you were here a few days ago?

Violet: I wasn't taking my medications, and I am hearing voices telling to kill myself.

Clinician: Are you having any thoughts of killing or hurting someone else?

Violet: No.

Clinician: Have you engaged in any kind of self-harm or self-injury?

Violet: No.

Clinician: Are you seeing anything that others would not say is there or you know isn't really there?

Violet: No.

Clinician: Do you feel paranoid that others are out to get you?

Violet: Yes.

Clinician: What day is it today?

Violet: Thursday.

Clinician: What are we doing?

Violet: Getting me into the hospital! How much longer is this going to take?

Clinician: For the record, what is your name?

Violet: I'm sick and detoxing!

Clinician: Ms. Violet, this is going to take about ten minutes. I need you to understand that you just left here four days ago, and we must have good information to justify you getting readmitted so soon. So, moving on. How much did you drink in the past twenty-four hours?

Violet: I don't know, five beers?

Clinician: What size beers?

Violet: Twenty-fours.

Clinician: We have it on record that you first used weed at age eighteen. When was the last time you used it?

Violet: Today.

Clinician: How much?

Violet: A hit on someone's joint.

Clinician: We know you first used cocaine at age thirty. When was the last time you used it?

Violet: Today and yesterday.

Clinician: How did you use it?

Violet: I smoked it.

Clinician: We know you first used meth at age forty. When was the last time you used it.

Violet: I haven't.

Clinician: So, you haven't used it in the last four days?

Violet: I never used it.

Clinician: Okay, since you were last here have you used heroin, LSD, acid, or shrooms?

Violet: Never.

Clinician: When was the last time you did benzos off the street?

Violet: Not in a long time.

Clinician: When was the last time you did spice or K2?

Violet: Months.

Clinician: Taken anyone else's pills?

Violet: No. This is taking too long.

Clinician: Ms. Violet, I have taken less than five minutes and I need five more. Are you going through any detox symptoms right now?

Violet: No.

Clinician: When was the last time you took your medications?

Violet: I don't know. I gotta go lay down.

Clinician: Moving onto other subjects. What was your sleep last night like?

Violet: Five hours.

Clinician: Your appetite: good, fair, or poor?

Violet: Good. I'm hungry.

Clinician: When was the last time you were able to get a bath or brush your teeth?

Violet: Three days.

Clinician: Do you feel helpless like you can't do anything right?

Violet: No. Now when are you done?

Clinician: About four more minutes. Do you feel hopeless like nothing good is going to happen to you?

Violent: No.

Clinician: I know that you have hypertension and high cholesterol. Have you been told you have any new medical issues in the last four days?

Violet: No.

Clinician: I have that you are allergic to sulfa drugs and shellfish. Have you been told you have any new allergies?

Violet: No.

Clinician: This is the sexual history section. I have previous information that you identify as bisexual and your pronouns are she/her. Do you consider yourself to have any new problems of a sexual nature that bother you?

Violet: No.

Clinician: This is none of my personal business, but they want to know if you consider yourself to be sexually active.

Violet: Yes.

Clinician: Do you practice safe sex?

Violet: No.

Clinician: Moving on, the record has that you were physically and sexually abused as a child by a family member, and a boyfriend had beaten you up. You also were neglected as a child. Have you been through any new abuse?

Violet: I don't want to talk about it.

Clinician: Two more questions. Have you been to any other hospital or therapy appointment in the last four days?

Violet: No.

Clinician: Okay: last question. Is there anyone who is supportive to you out in the community? Family or friends?

Violet: I ain't got nobody.

Clinician: Okay, Ms. Violet. I'm done. I'll give your doctor a call and get you a bed.

CONCLUDING THOUGHTS

High utilizers are a clinical challenge that this chapter sought to explain and suggest strategies in completing a successful assessment and prior authorization. It is natural to have countertransference toward many of them when they come in again and again and demonstrate savvy entitlement by which they may try to boss around the assessment clinician.

The matter of the high utilizer is a complex problem that is easy to dwell upon. High utilizers may be addicts, medication-non-compliant individuals with schizophrenia or bipolar disorder, personality disordered, or a combination of the three. They are survivors with a certain sense of resiliency despite their demonstrated inability to function like an average person in society. While some high utilizers (if they are willing to talk) can tell a series of tragedies and hardships, it can get "old," and it is logical to ask when the patient's problems started becoming their own responsibility. The high utilizer's irresponsibility especially shows in repeated failure to follow through with discharge recommendations.

In combination with the observed irresponsibility, many high utilizers can be rude, threatening, demanding, and may know the interview questions better than the clinician. The new clinician can feel intimidated by the high utilizer. In an ironic sense, as part of the resiliency and survivorship, high utilizers have invested time and energy in learning what it takes to get into the hospital, and that includes intimidating hospital staff. Furthermore, many high utilizers lie or avoid facts that the clinician can catch from chart review.[28] The limit to empathy and sympathy can quickly be reached in these cases, and the clinician's emotion can readily cross over into countertransference.

Even though countertransference is the natural tendency, the clinician still must compartmentalize feelings and provide a professional service to the patient. The development of such a professional attitude or mindset toward the high utilizer is a process that includes mastering the challenge of getting the interview done and not personalizing the patient's behavior.

Not personalizing an aggressive high utilizer's behavior can include applying the transactional analysis concepts discussed in chapter 4. An angry and aggressive adult is an immature person who is not acting like an adult but like a child. Such high utilizers with anger management problems do not take responsibility for their own emotional regulation and make themselves out to be victims. When the clinician can avoid personalizing the high utilizer's anger, they can stay focused on the interview and can be more able to practice the modified boredom skill and get through as much as the interview as possible.

Avoiding personalization of the high utilizer's anger does not mean the clinician is avoiding empathy. It is appropriate to recognize and verbally acknowledge that the patient is angry ("I can see that you are angry") as a way of respect and it can "buy" a few more moments of interview time to get questions answered.

When the patient is a known high utilizer with a history of being difficult, it is possible to get an assessment that is satisfactorily thorough by going at a fast pace and prioritizing the questions to establish criteria. After getting the initial reason for presentation, much of the interview may consist of confirmatory type questions. The patient may still leave the interview to avoid answering questions about drug use and trauma, but a higher-quality assessment will be completed.

It may be possible to divert a high utilizer by a case management approach when the patient's obvious issue is homelessness. However, the admitting department policy may not provide for such activity and the high utilizer may still reject any such discussion and focus only on what is necessary to be admitted. In the end, diverting high utilizers should be up to hospital administrators and the clinician should not be rogue in independently acting to divert.

In the end, dealing with high utilizers is largely a skill set that takes time and practice to develop. The concepts in this chapter have been offered for a foundation of such a skill set.

NOTES

1. S. N. Vigod, P. A. Kurdyak, C. Dennis, T. Leszcz, V. Taylor, D. M. Blumberger, and D. P. Seitz, 2013, "Transitional interventions to reduce early psychiatric readmissions in adults: Systematic review," *The British Journal of Psychiatry, 202*: 187–94.
2. The matter of child and adolescent high utilizers is generally a 1) family dysfunction issue or 2) a foster care/child-welfare placement issue. There are children and youth considered to be violent and seriously disturbed who cannot be consistently managed at lower levels of foster care residential treatment and who are frequently hospitalized.

3. J. E. Hamilton, R. Suchting, D. S. Buck, A. Chesnokova, S. Das, M. Allen, and R. Y. Cho, 2021, "Determinants of high psychiatric utilization at a large urban safety-net hospital," *Journal of Health Care for the Poor and Underserved, 32*: 296–320.

4. D. B. Mautner, H. Pang, J. C. Brenner, J. A. Shea, K. S. Gross, R. Frasso, and C. C. Cannuscio, 2013, "Generating hypotheses about care needs of high utilizers: Lessons from patient interviews," *Population Health Management, 16*: S26–S33.

5. J. Jiang, M. S. Barrett, and M. Sheng, 2014, "Characteristics of hospital stays for non-elderly Medicaid super-utilizers," HCUP Statistical Brief #184, Healthcare Cost and Utilization Project, https://hcup-us.ahrq.gov/reports/statbriefs/sb184-Hospital-Stays-Medicaid-Super-Utilizers-2012.pdf.

6. The lack of viable family support itself is complex. The family may have ostracized the patient due to behavior and/or addiction. The family members themselves may be unstable due to addiction or mental illness. The family may lack financial resources to help the patient. Family members who were close to the patient may be deceased and the living ones have unknown whereabouts. Most of the time, high utilizers will be guarded about the details of their family and dismiss the question in the assessment interview. The information in this paragraph is based on the authors' anecdotal experience with high utilizers while working in the inpatient setting.

7. J. Wilson, 1987, *The truly disadvantaged: The inner city, the underclass, and public policy*, Chicago: University of Chicago Press

8. A. Primeau, T. G. Bowers, and XuXu, 2013, "Deinstitutionalization of the mentally ill: Evidence for transinstitutionalization from psychiatric hospitals to penal institutions," *Comprehensive Psychology, 2*.

9. C. Bundy, M. Schreiber, and M. Pascualy, 2014, "Discharging your patients who display contingency based suicidality: 6 steps," *Current Psychiatry, 13*: e1–e3; M. T. Lambert and J. Bonner, 1996, "Characteristics and six-month outcome of patients who use suicide threats to seek hospital admission," *Psychiatric Services, 47* (8): 871–73.

10. The high utilizers avoiding legal obligations frequently report that they are missing court dates after admission and ask for admission letters be sent to courts and community corrections.

11. Many high utilizers are antagonistic toward unit staff and instigate drama. The unit staff members with low emotional intelligence often react in countertransference and perpetuate the drama. The drama between the patient and staff further perpetuates and possibly escalates with further admissions.

12. Generalizing the behavior beyond the unit suggests that the worldview of many high utilizers is that of survival. Some of these high utilizers with personality disorder have a sense of perpetual crisis in which they control interactions by refusing to cooperate with and commit to discharge planning. This type of patient also refuses to say what their plan is going to be when they leave the hospital out of apparent control; to let the hospital know things is to give up what control they do have.

13. If the high utilizer is to maintain sobriety and succeed in rehab treatment, they need to be capable of managing their emotions, getting along with others, and

be compliant with the rules at rehabilitation facilities. Many high utilizers have been through multiple rehabs and have been banned from returning due to behavior.

14. It is the experience of the authors that this type of high utilizer (with a few exceptions) tends to have addiction issues and spends all their money on drugs and alcohol instead of necessities.

15. Managed care organizations have refused to issue a prior authorization for high utilizers and many psychiatrists have discharged the patient the next day

16. C. Bundy, M. Schreiber, and M. Pascualy, 2014, "Discharging your patients who display contingency based suicidality: 6 steps," *Current Psychiatry, 13*: e1–e3.

17. K. Hempstead, D. DeLia, J. C. Cantor, T. Nguyen, and J. Brenner, 2014, "The fragmentation of hospital use among a cohort of high utilizers: Implications for emerging care coordination strategies for patients with multiple chronic conditions," *Medical Care, 52*: S67–S74.

18. Insurance case managers will also call the inpatient social worker or utilization management department after admission and disclose the recent admissions and discharges, but it is too late for the assessment clinician to know for the assessment.

19. This is opposed to observable, vegetative symptoms that include flat affect, response to internal stimuli, and disorganized thought patterns. The matter of not attending to activities of daily living is a variable in this case that may be more related to lack of access to resources versus being a symptom of depression or psychosis.

20. If it is a long-distance telehealth assessment and there is a closer state/public hospital that accepts involuntary petitions, the authors consider it an appropriate option to petition a high utilizer to that facility. It is a more efficient use of public resources to send them to an alternative, closer facility.

21. Specific exclusion of a high utilizer should be spelled out in a written hospital memorandum. This is often in cases when the high utilizer has engaged in severe aggression or property damage to a unit. Also, the clinician should discuss with a designated supervisor or administrator that the patient presented again and the content of the assessment. The clinician should then document in the assessment the review steps that were taken with supervisors and administrators.

22. Behavioral health units within medical-surgical hospitals or psychiatric hospitals directly attached (who use the same national provider) number can draw payment from a different Medicare "bucket" of money. Most proprietary psychiatric hospitals are not attached to medical-surgical hospitals and cannot draw from that Medicare bucket. This is not intended to be a criticism of the proprietary hospitals, but the authors recognize their constraints and that many of them provide excellent service to their communities.

23. There are several factors in the patient's waiting time to go to the unit. The nurses could be in report or doing medication pass. It could be "shift change." Staff shortages also could lengthen medication pass. Unit staff may also have countertransference toward the high utilizer and one shift may delay the admission to the next shift.

24. A similar situation was when a high utilizer acted out to go to the unit because the patient wanted to get in the patient's lunch order for the next day. The high utilizer seemed to know the unit schedule in detail.

25. See vignette #7 in chapter 3.

26. The reality is that as part of the development process, clinicians may look to patients for approval as to how the interview went or personally judge themselves that they are to blame for the failed interview. The high utilizer therefore has an incidental position of emotional power over the clinician in these cases.

27. It may be factual that the previous clinician did not ask it because the patient left the last interview before it could be asked.

28. A common example is when a patient claims not to have had any medication in weeks, but the clinician can look in the medical record and see that the patient was just discharged earlier in the day and had taken medication. It is not worth confronting the patient on the lies. However, the clinician should document the discrepancy in the medical record.

Chapter 14

Concluding Thoughts

Learning and Appreciating the Value of Communication

I (David) started working part time in my hospital's admitting department as a side gig. The hospital had a desperate need for clinicians and was recruiting in-house for people to fill in on a part-time basis. After a one-hour presentation and watching another experienced clinician conduct an assessment, I was told that I could do the next one on my own and she did not need to watch me. It felt like a bungee jump, but I was intrepid enough to do it because my motto at the time was that "I do difficult things." I remember feeling lucky because it was not a complicated case, but I remember asking many questions as to what was next and my colleagues were helpful if not tolerant. I was happy to be there and determined to master doing admission assessments, but I also look back and remember all the turnover in that department because the job was overwhelming in part due to the intensity, a lack of training, and a lack of consistent supervision.

John and I worked together in this department, and we watched it evolve in its training regimen over the years, so new clinicians were given extensive training and improved job orientation (especially by John). While the job is still emotionally challenging, the orientation and training processes have meant reduced turnover and improved employee retention. We saw that not all agencies and hospitals have the luxury or resources to provide extensive training and orientation to clinicians and thus we set out to write this book.

This book is written first for the master's level assessment clinician who may be in one of those situations that John and I started in where there may not be much training or orientation on how to do admission and emergency assessments. While we have suggested some theories to understand common clinical situations, we have more so sought to be practical in providing interview techniques and strategies and illustrate how they are used in numerous vignettes based on personal experience. We admit that learning these techniques and strategies will take time, but John and I agree that we have created a reference resource that also can be consulted again and again.

As stated before, this book emanates from the tacit knowledge and actual work experience of the authors. It demonstrates use of the evidence-based Columbia Suicide Scale, but this is not necessarily an evidence-based practice book. There has not been a previous, discernable, published book that contains research findings about admission and emergency assessment nor has there been academic research focusing on this practice setting.

Furthermore, while we do not explicitly discuss it, we feel that our methods and principles show fidelity to the principles of trauma-informed care in that they show awareness of the inherent power imbalance in the interview. We observe that patients show emotional reactivity to the assessment questions because the questions can trigger trauma memories. We aim to show respect for patients and uphold their dignity given that the assessment interview can be a retraumatizing experience; it does not necessarily seek to build a therapeutic alliance and it has questions an outpatient therapist would take several sessions to ask.

We cannot help but reiterate here that we have faced the reality of aggressive patients "head on" in this book. While some pathological patients appear to know exactly what they are doing when they throw tantrums, escalated anger is best considered as indication that a patient is in distress or emotional crisis to the point of being unable to cope with the environment to the extent that their ability to maintain self-control is diminished or gone. Patient aggression is that behavioral aspect of psychiatric crisis that can be shocking if not traumatic the first several times a clinician witnesses it. The inability to manage their own reactions and the inability to develop a rational response to patient anger has contributed to the clinician turnover. The professional development process of working with aggressiveness and agitation in essence involves something akin to exposure therapy where a clinician moves from reacting with emotion to responding with rational responses. At the risk of sounding like one motivational speaker who shall remain nameless here, our strategy of modified boredom could be called a *neuro-linguistic programming script* that a clinician practices and masters to intervene and manage encounters with angry and aggressive patients.

JOHN'S EXPERIENCES

Just because we are confident with the modified boredom strategy, we cannot diminish the need for clinicians to be mindful of safety for themselves, the patient, and others in the admitting department. At the end of the day, attempting to ensure no harm to anyone during the assessment process is the desired outcome. Communication with your colleagues and security personnel is key in maintaining safety. In the context of a learning process, I (John) personally once experienced a safety concern in which an adult female patient at a psychiatric hospital was reported by another patient to have a razor blade on her. I approached the individual who was unwilling to give up the contraband. I asked if she would speak with me in an assessment room to at least separate her from other patients and guests. Upon reaching the room, she ran to a corner and put the blade to her wrist. I instructed her to remain still and not cut herself. She began to cut her wrist at which time I immediately put her in a crisis management hold and a clinician passing by the doorway came in and removed the weapon from her hand. As I reflected on the event, in hindsight it I felt like I took the correct safety measures when in fact I now realize employing the assistance of at least one colleague or security officer may have assisted in the situation possibly making it safer; it increased my learning curve.

Furthermore, with respect to the learning process, I (John) was once sent to a medical-surgical hospital to evaluate a sixty-eight-year-old female admitted for surgery performed under anesthesia, who was experiencing psychosis. This individual evidenced paranoia, delusions, and hallucinations, and could not recognize family members with her; these were all new symptoms she had not previously exhibited. Upon arrival, I spoke with the attending physician whom I asked several questions to ascertain the origin of the psychosis that included the following:

- Did the patient possibly have a urinary tract infection?
- Was the toxicology screen positive for illicit drugs?
- Was there a family history of schizophrenia?

I then asked the patient and her accompanying family the following:

- Had the patient been experiencing insomnia or sleep deprivation?
- Were there any new life events such as
    - starting a new medication?
    - a traumatic event or a head injury?
    - a recent allergic reaction?

I explained the situation to the next psychiatrist on rotation. The psychiatrist educated me that older adults who had been given anesthetics can temporarily experience psychosis until the medication wears off. With this new learning, I stopped an unnecessary psychiatric admission and relayed the recommendation that the medical team should observe the patient for the next few hours in which time the symptoms would be resolved.

This situation taught me that the learning process in conducting assessments takes time. However, a clinician can significantly accelerate learning by slowing down their thinking with a questioning attitude and communicating with the all-available resources to assess what is going on and the next steps to take in the patient's well-being.

As far as suicide assessment and staffing with doctors being a learning process, I once knew a clinician who evaluated a high utilizer patient who had been discharged the day before but reported suicidal thoughts with a plan. The physician referred the patient to outpatient services. After being escorted from the hospital, the patient immediately went and laid down in the middle of the road and was admitted anyway that night after being brought back by the police. This event reminds us that assessment is not a pedestrian role requiring the clinician to ascertain the severity of a patient's suicidal ideation and advocate for patients to get the appropriate level of care.

On the other hand, sometimes a clinician has to say "no" and be the direct object of the anger and guilt trips from patients, their families, and any other stakeholders who have an emotional interest in the patient getting admitted. I had to tell a patient and his family that he was not going to be admitted despite it being what they wanted. The family's hostile expression of anger shook me up and made me question if I made the right assessment. I ruminated on the details and repeatedly concluded that the patient did not meet criteria for inpatient. A colleague noticing my angst said to me, "Our role is not to make patients happy. We are to provide a professional evaluation and make an appropriate referral."

On the other hand, a thorough explanation about the referral may reduce the likelihood of escalation. I (John) had a time when I was training a new clinician who referred an adolescent to the outpatient program and the patient's mother was upset that he was not going to be admitted to inpatient. The trainee asked me for help. I said we need to speak with the minor's mother about

- why the outpatient program referral was appropriate,
- what the program would offer,
- how he would benefit from it, and
- the mom's emergency recourse if her son's behavior were to worsen.

The extra communication was sufficient to calm the patient's mother.

Good communication (which can mean using ordinary words as opposed to clinical jargon) is also crucial for patient safety. In another training situation, a new clinician was assessing a patient for alcohol and drug withdrawal. The clinician asked the patient if he had ever experienced "delirium tremens or withdrawal seizures." The puzzled patient answered "No." At the end of the assessment, I stepped in and asked the patient if he knew what delirium tremens or withdrawal seizures were, to which he also answered "No." I then gave an explanation, and the patient related that his wife had told him he was like that in the past. He just did not know what those symptoms were called, and in that occasion the extra communication was potentially lifesaving.

Good communication skills also apply to seeking prior authorization with insurance companies. On countless occasions, insurance reviewers have attempted to get me to change my inpatient recommendation to a lower level of care such as intensive outpatient. At times it seemed that the insurance reviewer was arguing with me and debating me, and the situation necessitated defending the clinical decision by explaining the criteria used for inpatient admission. As discussed in chapter 12, the confidence and language to communicate during prior authorizations will come with time and practice.

DAVID'S EXPERIENCE

In keeping with John's theme of communication, my (David) one story to tell has to do with communicating with collateral sources prior to evaluations. It was in the early days of this new thing called telehealth, and I was to interview a female patient at a medical-surgical emergency department across town. I talked to one of the staff at the remote emergency room to get the patient in front of the camera and log in to the system, but not the nurse whom I should have talked to before the interview. The interview went something like this:

Me: Hello, ma'am. My name is David. I'm going to do your assessment. Why are you here?

Patient: I have a pain in my vagina.

Me: Ma'am, why else are you here?

Patient: I have a pain in my vagina.

Me: Ma'am, I'm a mental health clinician. Why do they have you talking to me?

Patient: Well sir, I have a pain in my vagina.

The patient plainly and flatly repeated the "pain in my vagina" line throughout the whole interview as a tangential answer to multiple questions. I was eventually able to get her to talk more about mental health issues that included she had previously had been at another hospital's psychiatric unit and that she had stopped taking her antipsychotic medication.

After I made it through the interview, I did what I should have done in the first place. I called the remote emergency department back and talked with the patient's nurse who told me that the patient had presented with a complaint of severe vaginal pain and had threatened that if they did not do something about it, she would go out into the parking lot and shoot herself. The physician put the patient on a seventy-two-hour hold and then referred her for an assessment. If I had known that information by talking to the nurse, I would have been effective in redirecting the patient to talk about the suicidal ideation and not her vaginal pain.

The lesson struck deeply for a while because while the word "vagina" is a frank, anatomical term that can be legally uttered on television and radio without repercussion from the Federal Communications Commission, it is not used in normal, polite human conversation. The sheer mention of the word often elicits responses of discomfort that the late John Bradshaw called in many of his works as "healthy shame."

So, in my healthy shame (also known as embarrassment in this case), I found myself having to repeat the word vagina multiple times to doctors, nurses, and the eventual insurance reviewer (to the snickers of my colleagues in the office). The first doctor on the rotation did not want the case. Luckily, the next doctor sounded amused by the story, took the case, and did not ask any further questions. The experience of healthy shame taught me to be sure to get solid collateral information from the referral source before I do telehealth assessments.

I cannot end this chapter with that story, so I will conclude to say that while I have had my moments of learning and humility like discussed earlier, conducting admission and emergency assessments has been a wonderful, fulfilling opportunity. It has exposed me to multiple clinical situations that challenged my critical thinking and emotional intelligence skills. That in turn improved my clinical skills as a therapist. While there have been crisis-filled shifts that drained me, there also have been many times where I left feeling honored to help people in their hours of crisis get to safety. The psychiatric hospital is a place of stigma, and going there in crisis adds an extra level of trepidation. My experience has taught me that a knowledgeable, accepting assessment clinician is able to do much everyday and ordinary good for the people in need who come through the door. While not always easy, this work has been a true calling or vocation for me. I have been grateful to be an assessment clinician and as such we hope that this book is a useful tool that not only helps readers learn how to do this work but also feel the satisfaction of doing it.

References

American Psychiatric Association. (2022). *Diagnostic and statistical manual of mental disorders* (fifth edition). American Psychiatric Association.

Beck, A. T. (1976). *Cognitive therapy and the emotional disorders*. International Universities Press.

Berman, A. C., and Chutka, D. (2016). Assessing effective physician-patient communication skills: "Are you listening to me, doc?" *Korean Journal of Medical Education, 28*(2): 243–49.

Berne, E. (1964). *Games people play*. Ballantine Books.

Bernstein, A. J. (2013). *Emotional vampires at work: Dealing with bosses and coworkers who drain you dry*. McGraw Hill Education.

Bundy, C., Schreiber, M., and Pascualy, M. (2014). Discharging your patients who display contingency based suicidality: 6 steps. *Current Psychiatry, 13*: e1–e3.

Gilliland, B. E., and James, R. K. (2016). *Crisis intervention strategies* (eighth edition). Cengage Learning.

Hadziabdic, E., and Hjelm, K. (2013). Working with interpreters: Practical advice for use of an interpreter in healthcare. *International Journal of Evidence-Based Healthcare, 11*: 69–76.

Haley, J. (1973). *Uncommon therapy: The psychiatric techniques of Milton H. Erickson, M.D.* W. W. Norton.

Hempstead, K., DeLia, D., Cantor, J. C., Nguyen, T., and Brenner, J. (2014). The fragmentation of hospital use among a cohort of high utilizers: Implications for emerging care coordination strategies for patients with multiple chronic conditions. *Medical Care, 52*: S67–S74.

Hietanen, J. K. (2018). Affective eye contact: An integrative review. *Frontiers in Psychology, 9*: 1587.

Houvenagle, D. (2015). *Clinicians guide to partial hospitalization and intensive outpatient practice*. Springer.

Hufford, R. (2001). Alcohol and suicidal behavior. *Clinical Psychology Review, 21*: 797–811. See also Cherpitel, C. J., Borges, G. L., and Wilcox, H. C. (2004). Acute alcohol use and suicidal behavior: A review of the literature. *Alcohol Clinical and Experimental Research,* (5 Suppl): 18S–28S.

Karpman, S. B. (2014). *A game free life. The definitive book on the drama triangle and compassion triangle by the originator and author. The new transactional analysis of intimacy, openness, and happiness.* Drama Triangle Publications.

Laffer, A. B. (2004). The Laffer curve: Past, present and future. Article 1765, The Heritage Foundation Publications.

Lambert, M. T., and Bonner, J. (1996). Characteristics and six-month outcome of patients who use suicide threats to seek hospital admission. *Psychiatric Services, 47*(8): 871–73.

Maslow, A. H. (1943). A theory of human motivation. *Psychological Review, 50*(4): 430–37.

Nápoles, A. M., Santoyo-Olsson, J., Karliner, L. S., Gregorich, S. E., and Pérez-Stable, E. J. (2015). Inaccurate language interpretation and its clinical significance in the medical encounters of Spanish-speaking Latinos. *Medical Care, 53*(11), 940–47.

McNiel, D. E. (1998). Empirically based clinical evaluation and management of the potentially violent patient. In P. M. Kleespies (Ed.), *Emergencies in mental health practice: Evaluation and management* (pp. 95–116). Guilford Press.

McNiel, D. E., Binder, R. L., and Greenfield, T. K. (1988). Predictors of violence in civilly committed acute psychiatric patients. *American Journal of Psychiatry, 145*: 965–70.

Monahan, J. (1981). *The clinical prediction of violent behavior.* National Institute of Mental Health.

Posner, K., Brown, G. K., Stanley, B., Brent, D. A., Yershova, K. V., Oquendo, M. A., Currier, G. W., Melvin, G. A., Greenhill, L., Shen, S. and Mann, J. (2011). The Columbia–suicide severity rating scale: Initial validity and internal consistency findings from three multisite studies with adolescents and adults. *American Journal of Psychiatry, 168*: 1266–77.

Primeau, A., Bowers, T. G., and XuXu. (2013). Deinstitutionalization of the mentally ill: Evidence for transinstitutionalization from psychiatric hospitals to penal institutions. *Comprehensive Psychology, 2.*

Prochaska, J. O., and Norcross, J. C. (2001). Stages of change. *Psychotherapy: Theory, Research, Practice, Training, 38*(4): 443–48.

Quan, K. (2011). *The high costs of language barriers in medical malpractice.* University of California-Berkley.

Steinhoff, A., Ribeaud, D., Kupferschmid, S., Raible-Destan, N., Quednow, B. B., Hepp, U., Eisner, M., and Shanahan, L. (2021). Self-injury from early adolescence to early adulthood: Age-related course, recurrence, and services use in males and females from the community. *European Child & Adolescent Psychiatry, 30*: 937–51.

Walker, L. (1979). *The battered woman.* Harper & Row.

Wesson, D. R., and Ling, W. (2003). The clinical opiate withdrawal scale (COWS). *Journal of Psychoactive Drugs, 35*(2): 253–59.

Index

About the Authors

David Houvenagle earned his bachelor's degree from Iowa State University. He has master's degrees from Bethel University–Minnesota (master of divinity) and the Carver School of Church Social Work–Southern Baptist Theological Seminary (master of social work). He earned his PhD in urban and public affairs from the University of Louisville. He is a board-approved LCSW, clinical supervisor, in the state of Kentucky. He has thirty years of professional experience in outpatient, partial hospitalization, intensive outpatient, inpatient hospitalization, and assessment settings. His previous published works include *Local Healthcare Politics: Louisville's Growth Machine 1947–2007* and *Clinician's Guide to Partial Hospitalization and Intensive Outpatient Practice*. (For the record, the name is pronounced HOH-veh-nay-guhl, or think Santa Claus on a bucking bronco . . . Santa goes "ho" and the horse goes "nay.")

John Schmanski, M.Ed., LPC, is a behavioral health case manager for an insurance company. He earned his bachelor's degree from Saint John's University/College of Saint Benedict and his master's of education from the University of Louisville. He has experience in inpatient and outpatient mental health settings. His experience in the behavioral health field spans fifteen years. As an assessment clinician at a psychiatric hospital, he evaluated patients for more than a decade and trained novice clinicians. (For the record, the name is pronounced shah-MAN-ski.)

www.ingramcontent.com/pod-product-compliance
Ingram Content Group UK Ltd.
Pitfield, Milton Keynes, MK11 3LW, UK
UKHW020056061026
476234UK00008B/122